Fitness
Through
Aerobics & Step Training

SECOND EDITION

Karen S. Mazzeo
Bowling Green State University

Morton Publishing Company
925 West Kenyon Avenue, Unit 12
Englewood, Colorado 80110

Typography by Ash Street Typecrafters, Inc., Englewood, Colorado
Editing by Carolyn Acheson, Aurora, Colorado
Cover Design by Bob Schram, Bookends, Inc., Boulder, Colorado
Cover Photo and Interior Photography by Jeffrey L. Hall Photography, Haskins, Ohio

CONTENTS

To the light of my life —
my best friend and husband
for these 30-plus years,

Richard A Mazzeo

Thank you for your constant support
regarding all the "hats" I wear —
writing, consulting, and teaching.
Your magic ingredients are patience and humor!

KSM

ACKNOWLEDGMENTS

Special appreciation to the following individuals who have shared
their time and superior talents in this endeavor:

Tobi Adams	Peter Holmes	Holly Naro
Steve Albrecht	Ruth Horton	Angela Peters
Laura Ware Babbitt	Virnette D. House	Dr. Bernard Rabin
Todd Belknap	Carin Peirce Johnson	Jane Rutter
Stephen I. Block	Vanya C. Jones	Joanne Saliger
Dr. Richard W. Bowers	Anthony 'Tony' Kaufman	Carrie Robinson Sanderson
Dr. Kathy Browder	Traci L. Kelly	Vivian Smallwood
Angie Carlucci	Cheryl Kirk, R.D., L.D.	Jennine Trotter
Jodi Cunningham	Tammy Kime-Sheets, R.D., L.D.	Harry Tyson
Dr. Lynn Darby	Lauren M. Mangili	John Virostek
Amy Marie Fondroy	Jen Marsick	Darlene Whipple
Sarah Foster	Mary Beth Mazzeo	Dan Youst
Philip H. Goldstein	Richard A. Mazzeo	
Jeffery L. Hall	Douglas N. Morton	

Appreciation to the following for granting permission
to use copyrighted materials:

Kenneth Cooper, M.D., M.P.H., and Bantam/Doubleday/Dell
Oregon Dairy Council
Werner W. K. Hoeger, Ph.D., and Morton Publishing Company

A special thank you to the following, for facility usage and equipment:

Dr. Mary Ann Roberton, Director, School Of Health, Physical Education, & Recreation,
Bowling Green State University, Bowling Green, OH
Kaufman's Downtown Restaurant, Bowling Green, Ohio
SPRI Products, Inc., Buffalo Grove, IL (1–800–222–7774) for rubber resistance bands, tubing, & shirts.

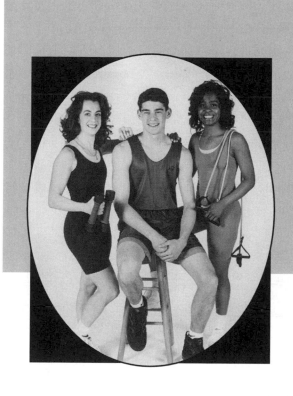

Introduction

Fitness Through Aerobics & Step Training and *Aerobics: The Way To Fitness* both have been updated and now are combined into this one text: *Fitness Through Aerobics and Step Training, Second Edition.*

This book presents the latest fitness research available, through both its descriptions and illustrations. It assists individuals like yourself, who are taking courses in physical fitness, to understand the principles and techniques involved in aerobic exercise — dance, step training, and fitness walking — and also to understand how to structure a complete physical and mental training program that will work for you, for a lifetime.

The aerobic fitness activities just mentioned — aerobic dance (also called aerobics), step training (which uses a 4"–12" step bench), and fitness walking (done at a pace equal to 14–20 minutes per mile) — are three of the most popular methods for achieving and maintaining physical fitness. Individually and collectively these aerobic exercise options have become extremely popular with fitness enthusiasts over the past several decades, and fitness industry professionals consider them as three important ways to achieve long-term adherence to fitness.

To provide a solid base from which to begin making your physical fitness choices, Chapter 1 gets you started thinking "fitness" by offering you the chance to make a personal commitment to fitness, followed by the definitions, necessary criteria, key principles and objectives, initial skills of monitoring various heart rates, and possible alternatives necessary to begin developing your own lifetime fitness program. You're encouraged to keep a Fitness Journal throughout the course, with a sample entry located in Chapter 15.

Chapter 2 provides the means to individualize your program according to your current or future needs, wants, and goals. It includes a discussion on motivation, its three component parts, plus details, examples, and suggestions on how to empower yourself if you're not motivated to do something. You're given the option of greatly improving your motivation by updating your "self talk," a key to your long-range attitude concerning fitness. Concluding this chapter are four steps for setting powerful goals. You now are ready and are given the opportunity to set specific goals for yourself, throughout every succeeding chapter in the book.

All physical fitness programs must be built upon a foundation of safety and on the needs and concerns that arise from both a preventive standpoint and after the fact. Chapter 3 first sets forth possible program challenges, or problem areas and then gives solutions to consider. Chapter 4 continues the safety theme with body positions to consider in conjunction with the exercise modalities in which you choose to engage. It emphasizes proper postural alignment, as good positioning, especially of the spine and joints, underlies all physical movement. This chapter, therefore, is paramount and marks the point where the techniques of your fitness program must begin.

Chapter 5 establishes where you are today, through testing procedures that enable you to describe your starting point. Then you will be able to establish specific goals and have a measured standard against which to monitor your progress continually throughout the course.

New to this *Second Edition* is the layout of the four key program segments of any total fitness course. Chapter 6 details the principles and techniques involved in the first program segment — the warm-up — to proceed any form of exercise.

Chapters 7, 8, and 9 present the options of aerobics, step training, and fitness walking, respectively. Chapter 7 presents the principles of building, sustaining, and lowering heart rate intensity via the kinds of impact and other criteria. This chapter contains a wealth of basic aerobics step and gesture techniques, and how to apply creative variation to these techniques.

Chapter 8 presents the aerobic exercise modality of step (bench) training. The principles and basic techniques for safe, efficient, and varied movement are detailed here. Included are the directional approaches, steps, patterns, and variations possible, concluding with the opportunity to create your own patterns.

The exercise movements in Chapters 6, 7, and 8 are all photographed using a "mirrored" method. A movement described and visualized as using the left foot/arm/side of the body is actually the right foot/arm/side of the model (see Figure I.1). Thus, you do not have to reverse the direction of what is pictured and what you perform. You simply do the movement on the same side of the body as you see it photographed and described.

Chapter 9 concludes the aerobic exercise modality options presented in this text with fitness walking and a brief discussion of rope jumping. With so many aerobic possibilities from which to choose, lifetime adherence to exercise becomes more of a reality for participants in the course.

Chapter 10 targets the third program segment, strength training. Given along with the principles are suggestions on how to apply those principles in any aerobic modality — aerobic-dance only, step training, fitness walking, or any combination of these. The techniques use a variety of resistance — your

FIGURE I.1   **Mirrored Method of Photography**

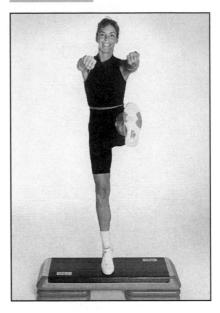

Step up *left*, kick *right* leg, waist high.

own weight as the resistance, hand-held weights, and various resistance bands and tubing, alone or in conjunction with the bench.

Chapter 11 concludes the presentation of the four key program segments with the principles and techniques for cooling down and stretching properly to increase flexibility.

The principles of stress management, with accompanying relaxation techniques, are presented in Chapter 12. Understanding creative ways to rejuvenate your mental and physical energy immediately following exercise is the revitalizing touch needed in physical fitness programs.

Chapter 13 focuses on the intake of energy — your diet and current nutritional concerns. Monitoring food and beverage intake for one week is encouraged with assessments provided in Chapter 15. A discussion of body image, assessment of your body composition, and the weight wellness mindset provides the foundation for positive weight management found in Chapter 14.

Chapter 15 concludes by offering you the opportunity to evaluate your progress, review the goals you've set, celebrate any goals already achieved, post-test any portions of the course you choose, and establish short-, medium-, or long-term goals toward which to strive daily.

> *You alone are the Captain of your ship*
> *You alone control the choices*
> *No one, and nothing else*
> *can do it for you . . .*

Student Information Profile

Please fill in the following information, remove from the textbook, and give to your instructor:

Name _____ Rank: F / So / J / S / Grad / Other

Address _____ Phone _____

Student I.D. No. _____ Age _____ Height _____ Weight _____ Ideal Weight _____

Rate Your Fitness Level: SUPERIOR / EXCELLENT / GOOD / FAIR / POOR / VERY POOR—PRE

                              SUPERIOR / EXCELLENT / GOOD / FAIR / POOR / VERY POOR—POST

Previous class or instruction in course:_____

Sports in which you participate/enjoy weekly: _____

Reason(s) for taking course: _____

Did anyone recommend this course or instructor? _____

If so, whom? _____

Physical limitations: _____

Activity that you would especially like instructor to cover: _____

Heart rate: Resting _____ Training Zone _____ – _____

List any drug you take (that may alter your heart rate): _____

Do you desire to: (circle) Gain lean weight / Lose fat weight / Stay same

Do you smoke? _____ If so, number of cigarettes per day: _____

Rate your alcohol consumption: Never/Daily/Other/ _____

List interest in music, favorite song, favorite artist: _____

Other interests:_____

If age 35 or older, or have specific limitation: I have my doctor's written permission to participate.

Doctor's name and phone number: _____

I have read and understand the responsibilities for participants and the instructor.

_____   _____
             Signature   Date

Student Physical Activity Readiness

Name _____

Address _____

Phone (Bus.) _____ (Home) _____ Age _____ Height _____ Weight _____

(**NOTE:** The purpose of this questionnaire is to serve as part of prescreening for both fitness testing and exercise participation. If you respond "Yes" to any question, your instructor will want to talk to you further.)

	YES	NO
1. Has your doctor ever said that you have heart trouble?	_____	_____
2. Do you frequently suffer from pain in your chest or heart, especially with exercise?	_____	_____
3. Do you often feel faint or have spells of severe dizziness? More so with exercise?	_____	_____
4. Has your doctor ever told you that you have high blood pressure?	_____	_____
5. Have you ever been told you have a heart murmur?	_____	_____
6. Has a doctor ever told you that you have a bone or joint problem such as arthritis that has been aggravated by exercise or might be made worse by exercise?	_____	_____
7. Do you have diabetes mellitus?	_____	_____
8. Are you over age 35 and unaccustomed to vigorous exercise?	_____	_____
9. Are you taking any medications or other drugs that might alter your response to exercise?	_____	_____
10. Are you pregnant?	_____	_____
11. Are you a smoker?	_____	_____
12. Have you recently had surgery, are you obese, or do you have special limitations?	_____	_____
13. Do you have an at-risk cholesterol reading?	_____	_____
14. Do you have an abnormal resting ECG?	_____	_____
15. Do you have any family history of coronary disease, before or by age 50?	_____	_____
16. Is there a good physical reason not mentioned here why you should not follow an activity program?	_____	_____

If you answered YES to any question, please provide a brief explanation (use separate sheet if necessary).

I have answered the above questions to the best of my knowledge.

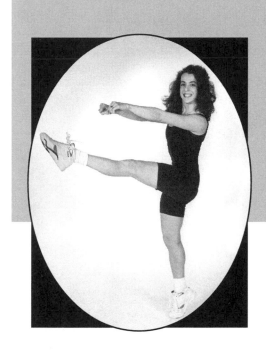

Aerobic Exercise: The Way to Fitness

PHYSICAL FITNESS: A CHOICE

Fitness is one of life's positive choices. By making the decision to engage in the physical fitness activities that follow — aerobics, step training, fitness walking, strength and endurance training, and flexibility training — you've taken the important first initiative toward achieving a meaningful, active, and healthy lifestyle. Incorporating a variety of regular physical activity into your life provides the foundation and basis for a long life of quality rather than just existing and "putting in time" in life.

The "use it or lose it" philosophy is a core belief that you must accept if true fitness is the goal you seek. This text will provide you with the knowledge base from which to "use it" wisely — safely, efficiently, timely. Knowledge is not power, though. The *application* of knowledge is power, and the all-important application of knowledge rests on your shoulders, in your hands, and through your feet. It must be triggered by your mind and fueled by your will. Ideas to facilitate this triggering and fueling will be given throughout every chapter of the text so you will develop the mental training along with the physical conditioning.

Achieving physical fitness requires a commitment and dedication to personal excellence. Shortcuts are few, but pleasurable alternatives are many.

Once you have achieved physical fitness, you must maintain your fitness for a lifetime. Fitness is a journey — a continual process — not just one destination. Make a personal commitment to fitness at the onset of this course (see form in Chapter 15). Maintaining fitness is a lot easier than achieving it initially, though you will also discover that the less physically fit you are, the longer you will take to become fit.

> The total physical fitness journey requires:
>
> ● making a commitment to fitness
> ● seeking valid information
> ● establishing your starting points
> ● setting reasonable and challenging goals
> ● monitoring your daily progress
> ● making self-disciplined choices continually

The learning process begins by first understanding the basics, which requires a common language that communicates the essentials of achieving fitness. The process of learning and doing, and then achieving and maintaining, fitness for a lifetime is powerful and rewarding.

DEFINITIONS

Most simply stated, the term *aerobic* means *promoting the supply and use of oxygen*. All body cells require oxygen to exist. The body's demand for oxygen increases when you engage in vigorous activity that produces specific beneficial changes in the body. Aerobic, therefore, refers to *any exercise mode as long as certain basic criteria are met*.

Within the last decade the exercise mode entitled *aerobic dance*, generalized since then to the term *aerobic exercise dance*, has been abbreviated to the currently preferred term *aerobics*. Still, these terms are used interchangeably to mean the same activity. Again, *aerobic* is an adjective, and *aerobics* is the noun denoting a mode of activity.

HEALTHY LIFESTYLE CHOICES

Associated fitness behaviors that enhance the ability to perform well during physical conditioning workouts include eating nutritionally, maintaining proper body weight, relaxing, and getting an adequate amount of sleep. Without a balance in *biochemical functioning* — energy intake, energy expenditure, and energy rejuvenation — the positive effects and benefits of exercise will not occur. Each of these healthy lifestyle choices is introduced here, and expanded in later chapters.

Eating

To provide the fuel needed to produce the energy required for all aerobic exercise and to ensure proper body regulatory functions, growth, and repair, participants should eat a well-balanced diet that provides all the nutrients needed to stay well, to be able to perform well, and to maintain a proper weight.

Regarding how much to eat and the time of day for eating, food intake should generally follow a *25–50–25 rule:* 25% of intake for breakfast, 50% for lunch, and 25% for the evening meal. Incidentally, weight control is easier for those who exercise either before breakfast or 1½ hours after the heaviest meal of the day.[1]

Participants should refrain from eating for 1, or preferably 2, hours before participating in aerobic activity and, instead, eat afterward. In digesting food, an increased amount of blood and oxygen is needed in the digestive tract. With exercise as much as 100 times more oxygen is needed in the working muscles (arms and legs) than when at rest. The body has great difficulty increasing blood and oxygen to two major body systems at once.

Relaxing and Sleeping

Quality time should be set aside for reflective relaxation, along with adequate sleep. These are important restorative mechanisms. Aerobic exercise takes a great deal of energy, and the body's way of restoring energy is through relaxation and sleep, which help restore the ability to concentrate and to maintain a positive attitude. Physiologically, relaxation and sleep help by lowering both the body temperature and the heart rate, which in turn lower the body's demand for oxygen and nutrients, thereby conserving while restoring the body's supply of energy.

A TOTAL PHYSICAL FITNESS CONDITIONING PROGRAM

Total physical fitness is the *positive state of well-being allowing you enough strength and energy to participate in the full, active lifestyle of your choice*. According to the American Medical Association, it is "the general capacity to adapt favorably to physical effort. Individuals are physically fit when they are able to meet both the usual and unusual demands of daily life, safely and effectively without undue stress or exhaustion."

A total physical fitness conditioning program consists of five basic elements. This can be visualized by the fitness triangle, depicting three action components surrounding two underlying structural components, as shown in Figure 1.1.

1. *Aerobic fitness* (cardiovascular and respiratory)
2. *Flexibility* (ability to bend and stretch)
3. *Muscular strength and muscular endurance* (thickening muscle fiber mass to enable individuals to endure a heavier work load)
4. *Good posture* (holding body in proper position for safety and efficiency)
5. *Body composition* (maintaining proper fat-to-lean weight ratio).

FIGURE 1.1   Fitness Triangle

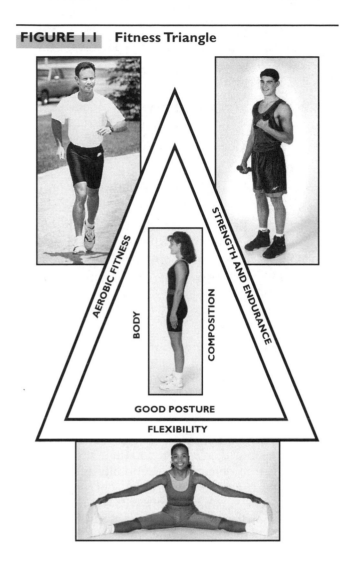

FIGURE 1.1   Fitness Triangle

more blood with each stroke, and with a more efficient stroke volume your heart can function with less effort. By getting your heart into condition, you may be practicing preventive medicine. You may be lessening the danger of a coronary heart attack 5, 10, 15, 20 years from now. And if you do have a heart attack, your chances of surviving are far greater if your heart, lungs, and blood vessels are in good condition.[2]

A person can exist without big, bulging muscles or without the perfect figure or with a head cold, but not very long without a good heart and lungs. Unfortunately, more than 40% of all people who have a first heart attack do not receive a second chance to change their habits or develop an aerobic program; they die.[3] And nearly half of all American deaths each year are attributed to heart-related diseases.[4] If only we could establish a living pattern priority early in life to counteract this overwhelming statistic!

Aerobic Fitness

A total, well-rounded fitness conditioning program should involve all five components. Because the sign of true fitness is the condition of the heart, blood vessels, and lungs, however, aerobic fitness is considered the most important component. By engaging in aerobic exercise-dance (or any other aerobic activity, such as step training), the heart gradually strengthens and develops a greater capacity to pump more oxygenated blood to the body with fewer contractions. Exercised hearts are stronger and beat slower.

Highly trained and conditioned endurance athletes have resting heart rates as low as 30 to 32 beats per minute, an admirably low rate. What actually happens is that with regular, stimulating exercise, the heart becomes a more efficient pump. It pumps

Flexibility

Flexibility is defined as *the functional range of motion of a given joint and its corresponding muscle groups.* The greater the range of movement, the more the muscles, tendons, and ligaments can flex or bend. Muscles are arranged in pairs. One muscle's ability to shorten or contract is related directly to the opposing muscle's length or stretch. Flexibility is maintained or increased by movement patterns that stretch the muscle slowly and progressively beyond its relaxed length. The stretch is performed to a point at which tension developing in the muscle is felt, but not to a point of pain.

Muscular Strength/ Muscular Endurance

Muscular strength is the *ability of a muscle to exert a force against a resistance.* Strength activities increase the amount of force that muscles can exert, or the amount of work that muscles can perform. Activities such as weight training can develop strength in the skeletal muscles.

Muscular endurance is the *ability of muscles to work strenuously for progressively longer periods* without fatigue. It is the capacity of a muscle to exert a force repeatedly, or to hold a static (still) contraction over time.

Muscular strength and endurance activities do not provide increased oxygen to condition the heart to function more efficiently.[5] Their primary target is skeletal muscle.

Good Posture/Good Positioning

Proper positioning of the body when performing any type of physical exertion promotes a safe and efficient workout. Once the basic mechanics are known and practiced, this fitness component becomes an integral part of every move.

Body Composition

An individual's total body weight is composed of fat weight and lean weight (fat-free weight). Keeping an appropriate ratio between these two weights is important for the entire body's best functioning and helps prevent obesity and its many health risks. This fitness component is managed by establishing a proper diet and exercise plan that provides for maintenance of ideal weight. If you aren't beginning your program at your ideal weight, you can consult the specific guidelines, within the physical exercise programs and the dietary eating plans, for establishing how to achieve your recommended ideal weight.

In summation, of the five components involved in developing a total physical fitness conditioning workout program (your *prescription exercise plan*), aerobic fitness training is considered the most important. The remainder of this chapter is devoted to a detailed look at the research and general principles recommended for you to follow, including modes of activity and monitoring techniques. Aerobic exercise modalities and techniques and the other four physical fitness components are explained more fully in later chapters.

AEROBIC FITNESS TRAINING

Training refers to muscle stimulation. Therefore, *aerobic training is any exercise that requires a steady supply of oxygen for an extended time and demands an uninterrupted work output from the muscles.*

Activities such as aerobics, step training, and fitness walking significantly increase the oxygen supply to all body parts, including the heart and the lungs, through continuous, rhythmic movement of large muscles and connective tissue. This type of movement conditions the body's oxygen transport system (heart, lungs, blood, and blood vessels) to process the use of oxygen more efficiently. This *efficiency in processing oxygen is called aerobic capacity* and depends on your ability to:

- Rapidly breathe large amounts of air.
- Forcefully deliver large volumes of blood.
- Effectively deliver oxygen to all parts of the body.

In short, one's aerobic capacity depends upon efficient lungs, a powerful heart, and a good vascular system. Because it reflects the conditions of these vital organs, *aerobic capacity is the best index (single measure) of overall physical fitness.*

Aerobic capacity is what is measured, quantified, and labeled in a physical fitness stress test, performed either in a laboratory (called a laboratory stress test) or on a premeasured distance such as a track (called a field stress test). You are given the opportunity to test your aerobic capacity in Chapter 5, using either method.

Progressive Overload Principle

Aerobic exercise dance, step training, fitness walking, or any aerobic activity conditions the heart muscle by strengthening it through a principle called *progressive overload*. Not only will the heart pump more blood with each beat, but it also will have longer rests between each beat, thereby lowering the pulse rate. Aerobic exercise overloads the heart by causing it to beat faster during a specific timeframe of the workout session, making a temporary high demand on the cardiorespiratory system. Over time, as you become more fit, the heart eventually adjusts to this temporary high demand, and soon it is able to do the same amount of work with less effort.

By overloading the heart with any vigorous aerobic exercise, your aerobic capacity increases and a desirable training effect can be achieved. The *training effect*, or total beneficial changes that usually occur, consists of:

- Stronger heart, sending more oxygenated blood to all tissues of the body.
- Production of more blood cells.
- Slower resting heart rate.
- Expanded blood vessels.
- Improved muscle tone.
- Lower blood pressure through improved circulation.
- Stronger respiratory muscles.

- Regulation of the release of adrenalin.
- Increased lung capacity.
- More regular elimination of solid wastes.
- Lower levels of fat found in blood.[6]
- Strengthening of muscles and skeleton to protect them from injury later in life.
- Deterring osteoporosis by increasing bone density.[7]
- Increased sensitivity to insulin and lowered blood sugar levels in mild, adult-onset diabetes.[8]
- Improvement in the way the body handles cholesterol, by increasing the proportion of blood cholesterol attached to high-density lipoprotein (HDL), a carrier molecule that keeps cholesterol from damaging artery walls.[9]

Aerobic Exercise Alternatives

Aerobic exercise options encompass all of the following:

- Aerobic exercise dance (aerobics)
- Bench/step training
- Cross-country skiing
- Cycling (including stationary cycling)

- Jogging/running
- Jumping rope
- Rowing
- Skating (ice/roller/in-line)
- Stair climbing
- Swimming
- Walking/hiking (moderate to fast pace-walk).

Aerobic Criteria

For the exercise to be labeled "aerobic," these exercise alternatives, collectively, must have several essential criteria (see Figure 1.2). The movements you do must meet the following criteria:

1. *They must use the large muscles of the body*[10] (arms and legs). Exercise gesture and step patterns found in aerobic exercise dance and bench step movements are excellent choices.

2. *They must be rhythmic.*[11] One-two-one-two, accompanied by a steady beat of music using either a fast or slow tempo, is suggested.

3. *They must be done a minimum of three sessions per week.*[12]

   - Four days a week or every other day is the suggested guideline.

FIGURE 1.2 **Five Aerobic Criteria**

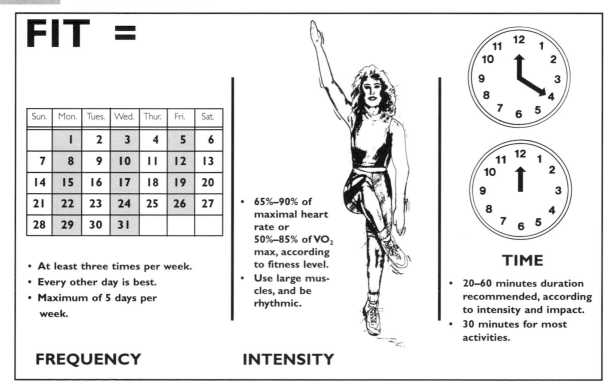

FIT =

Sun.	Mon.	Tues.	Wed.	Thur.	Fri.	Sat.
	1	2	3	4	5	6
7	8	9	10	11	12	13
14	15	16	17	18	19	20
21	22	23	24	25	26	27
28	29	30	31			

- At least three times per week.
- Every other day is best.
- Maximum of 5 days per week.

FREQUENCY

- 65%–90% of maximal heart rate or 50%–85% of VO_2 max, according to fitness level.
- Use large muscles, and be rhythmic.

INTENSITY

TIME

- 20–60 minutes duration recommended, according to intensity and impact.
- 30 minutes for most activities.

- Some key researchers recommend 5 days as a maximum. Beyond this, injuries to the musculoskeletal system from overuse are ten times more likely to occur. Novices to physical fitness conditioning need at least 2 days off per week.

- For those whose athletic status requires more workouts or days per week, *the body will reveal maximum frequency.* A sudden elevated resting heart rate in the morning signifies the day(s) not to work out. This is a built-in body signal, and it can be seen/heard/felt readily simply by monitoring the resting heart rate daily. Upon arising in the morning, this heart rate is monitored for one full minute.

4. *They must be done continuously for 20–60 minutes.*[13]

- Duration depends upon the intensity and the impact of the activity. (Both of these terms are explained later in full detail — intensity below and impact in Chapter 7.)

- Lower intensity and impact activities, such as fitness walking, should be done over a longer period (40–60 minutes).

- Because high-impact types of activity, such as running and jumping, generally cause significantly more debilitating injuries to exercisers, shorter workouts (20 minutes) are recommended.

5. *They must maintain the heart rate in a specific target heart rate training zone,* the individualized safe pace at which to work or exercise aerobically. This reflects intensity and is explained scientifically as one of the following:

- 65%–90% of your maximum heart rate or
- 50% to 85% of your maximum oxygen uptake, or heart rate reserve.[14]

Intensity

Frequency and time duration of workouts are easy to determine, but the amount of exertion (intensity) during the workout to keep it safe while making fitness gains continually can be more of a challenge to determine, especially for the novice. Intensity is measured or monitored in one of three ways:

- Finding your target heart rate (THR) training zone using the Karvonen formula. This is suggested for the novice.

- Using the Borg scale for ratings of perceived exertion (RPE), which shows a high correlation with heart rate and other metabolic parameters, according to American College of Sports Medicine (ACSM) guidelines. RPE monitoring is suggested for individuals who already have become accustomed to taking a heart rate pulse.

- Using the talk test. This easy and practical method is best used in conjunction with the THR and RPE for monitoring exercise intensity.

TARGET HEART RATE TRAINING ZONE

Taking Your Pulse To calculate appropriate exercise intensity using the target heart rate training zone method, you first must know how to take your pulse accurately. The pulse equals heartbeats per minute and can be felt and counted at one of six pulsation points. Select the area from which you can best obtain a pulse, using your index and second fingers. The two places most often used to count the pulse are the neck near the carotid artery and the wrist near the radial artery. Both are shown in Figure 1.3.

1. The carotid artery, located in the neck, is usually easy to find. Place your index and middle fingers below the point of your jawbone and slide downward an inch or so, pressing lightly. When you use the carotid artery pulse-monitoring method, make sure to apply light pressure, as

---

FIGURE 1.3

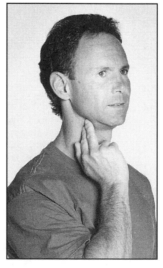 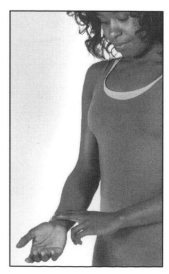

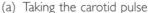

(a) Taking the carotid pulse   (b) the radial pulse

excessive pressure may cause the heart rate to slow down by a reflex action.

2. The radial artery extends up the wrist on the thumb side. Place your index and middle fingers just below the base of your thumb. Press lightly. Count the number of pulsations, or beats, for 60 seconds. The total is the number of heartbeats per minute. To count correctly, make sure you count each beat you feel.

Having gained the skill of pulse taking, you can establish your *resting heart rate*. This number is to be placed in the formula for establishing your target heart rate training zone.

Monitoring Resting Pulse Rate A true *resting heart rate* (RHR) is not taken in a class but, instead, when you have been at complete rest, preferably sleeping for several hours and upon awakening. Keep a clock or watch with a second hand next to your bed. When you awaken (without an alarm clock ring), take your pulse for 1 full minute and record that number as your RHR. Do this on five consecutive mornings, then determine an average (add all RHRs and divide by 5). This is a rather accurate determination of your resting heart rate.

Week I:

Day I: _____

Day 2: _____

Day 3: _____

Day 4: _____

Day 5: _____

Sum total:_____

÷ 5:_____ RHR

Unusual stress and illness (illness is a type of stress) sharply elevate the resting heart rate from previous readings.

Normally healthy individuals, therefore, should find a positive outlet for stress. Stress affects you even as you sleep (through a constant rapid heart rate), a time when the heart ideally should take a break and slow down for 6 to 8 hours.

One of the two visible signs of improvement in heart and lung fitness is a lower resting heart rate. Because the RHR is the basic thermometer of fitness,

after a 10- to 15-week aerobics course you and your classmates may experience:

● An average −3 heartbeats per minute resting heart rate decline.

● An average −10 heartbeats per minute by smokers who quit (or change their consumption significantly) during the course and as much as a −24 heartbeats per minute decline.[15]

Continue to monitor your RHR for the entire course on form provided in Chapter 15.

Determining Target Heart Rate Training Zone
Your average RHR figure is now placed in the formula for determining your target heart rate (THR) training zone (see Figure 1.4). The other variables figured into the formula are current *age* and *lifestyle*, represented as a percentage of maximum heart rate.

If you are:	Use:
● a nonathletic adult	50% to begin
● sedentary	60%–69%
● moderately active	70%–75%
● very active and well-trained	80%–85%

Record your age and the selected percentage range from above that describes your lifestyle. Figure the Karvonen equation. The result is your target heart rate, the safe exercise training zone for you.

Taking a Count After an Aerobic Interval As you begin an aerobic fitness program, you will want to monitor your pace several times during the workout hour so you can learn constant endurance pacing. Mentally remember your readings, and record them at the end of class on form provided in Chapter 15.

When you take a pulse rate during the learning process and find that your pace is *below* your established training zone, increase your intensity. If you have a pulse rate *higher* than your established training zone, lower your intensity.

To become familiar with your own response to various intensity levels so you can regulate yourself better, ask yourself, "How do I feel when I get this pulse?" Focus not only on your pulse count but also on what feelings and conditions the number relates to, so you can begin to recognize the signals your body sends. This also will help prepare you to use the RPE monitoring method of intensity, which, as you become a more advanced exerciser, will be a more practical method than counting your heartbeats per minute.

FIGURE 1.4 **How to Figure Your Target Heart Rate Training Zone**

Three basic factors enter into figuring your estimated safe exercise zone. These must be established first:

1. Current age:_____

2. How active is your lifestyle? _____% MHR.

   If you are: (Choose one and place on the line above:)

   ● Nonathletic adult: use 50% of your maximum heart rate.
   ● Sedentary: use 60%–69% of your maximum heart rate
     (but only for the first 2 or 3 weeks).
   ● Moderately physically active: use 70%–75% of your maximum heart rate.
   ● Active and well-trained: use 80%–85% of your maximum heart rate.

3. Your average resting heart rate (just figured): _____

Now place your numbers in the Karvonen formula:

A. 220   – _____ = _____**Estimated maximal heart rate (MHR)**
   (Index number)   **(Your age)**

B. _____ – _____ = _____
      MHR   **Resting HR**   **Heart Rate Reserve**

C. _____ × ._____ = _____ + **Resting HR** = _____*
 Heart Rate Reserve   **Lower end lifestyle**
              activity range (i.e. #2 above)

 _____ × ._____ = _____ + **Resting HR** = _____*
 Heart Rate Reserve   **Higher end lifestyle**
              activity range (i.e. #2 above)

RANGE

RANGE OF   _____*   This range is your estimated safe exercise zone. Keep your heart rate working in this range while you exercise aerobically for approximately 30 minutes of each session.

YOUR

TARGET   _____*   Refigure as you "age," as you can reclassify your lifestyle percentage, or as your resting heart rate declines markedly.

For example: Chris is 20 years old, a moderately active person (70%–75% range), with a resting heart rate of 62.

A. 220 – 20 = 200 MHR

B. 200 – 62 = 138 Heart rate reserve

C. 138 × .70 = 96 + 62 = 158*
   138 × .75 = 104 + 62 = 166*) Target heart rate training zone

If Chris keeps working (aerobically exercising) at the range of 158 to 166 heartbeats per minute, the heart would be working safely toward the training effect.

Continuing at a pace that is too intense will prove to be an *anaerobic* exercise program. *Anaerobic* activity is basically stop and start, in which the heart is not kept at a constant, steady pace for 20 to 60 minutes. Anaerobic describes an activity that requires all-out effort of short duration and does not utilize oxygen to produce energy. This type of exercise quickly uses up more oxygen than the body can take in while engaging in the exercise, causing an oxygen debt. This in turn causes lactic acids (waste products) to accumulate in the muscles, which leads to exhaustion.

Next, slow down, walk around, find your pulse, and count it for either 6 or 10 seconds. Each of these counts has been found to be a scientifically accurate measurement for aerobic activity pulse rates. Taking a timed count of greater than 10 seconds immediately after aerobic exercise will tend to be inaccurate because the heart rate slows down to a *recovery* pulse rapidly. You or your instructor will determine whether you will count for 6 or 10 seconds. Immediately following the aerobic exercise segment, count your pulse and multiply the number you get times 10 if using the 6-second count, or times 6 if using a 10-second count. *Each of these newly multiplied numbers will equal heartbeats per minute and hopefully will always be in your training zone.*

Taking a 6-second count is easy. All you do is add a zero to the pulse you feel, and record that number. You must begin and end exactly with a timer.

Table 1.1 lists target heart rate counts for individuals who wish to attain fitness using the ideal aerobic range for most people (60%–75% of heart rate reserve). Locate the column across the top that is closest to your age and the row down and left side reflecting a figure closest to your resting heart rate. The box where the column and row intersect is *your 10-second target heart rate training zone.*

As your cardiorespiratory system becomes more fit and efficient, work (exercise) will become easier, and you will have to increase the intensity of your activities. Techniques for increasing and decreasing the intensity of your workout will be explained in Chapters 7–11. By using the target heart rate training zone, you automatically compensate for increased fitness and still maintain the same training effect. Thus, your heart rate will increase during vigorous aerobic activity and should return to normal (pre-activity heart rate) within a short time after the workout. As a rule, the faster it slows down (recovers from exercise), the more physically fit you are, for recovery heart rate improvement is another indication of increased fitness level.

RATINGS OF PERCEIVED EXERTION: BORG SCALE

The second method for monitoring intensity utilizes the psychophysical Borg scale for ratings of

TABLE 1.1 **Target Heart Rate Training Zones***

| | | Your Age | | | | | | | | | | | | |
		15	20	25	30	35	40	45	50	55	60	65	70	75	80
Your average Resting Heart Rate per minute	90	27-29	26-29	26-28	25-28	25-27	24-26	23-26	23-25	22-24	22-24	21-23	21-22	20-22	20-21
	85	26-29	26-29	25-28	25-27	24-27	24-26	23-25	23-25	22-24	22-24	21-23	21-22	20-22	20-21
	80	26-29	25-28	25-28	24-27	24-26	23-26	23-25	22-25	22-24	21-23	21-23	20-22	20-21	19-21
	75	26-29	25-28	25-28	24-27	24-26	23-26	23-25	22-25	21-24	21-23	20-23	20-22	19-21	19-21
	70	25-29	25-28	24-27	24-27	23-26	23-25	22-25	22-24	21-24	21-24	20-22	20-22	19-21	19-20
	65	25-28	25-28	24-27	23-26	23-26	22-25	21-24	21-24	21-23	20-23	20-22	19-21	19-21	18-20
	60	25-28	24-28	24-27	23-26	23-26	22-25	21-24	21-24	20-23	20-22	19-22	19-21	18-21	18-20
	55	24-27	23-27	23-27	23-26	22-25	21-24	21-24	21-24	20-23	20-22	19-22	19-21	18-20	18-20
	50	24-28	23-27	23-26	22-26	22-25	21-25	21-24	20-23	20-23	19-22	19-21	18-21	18-20	17-20

*The numbers in the squares represent pulse beats counted in 10 seconds.

perceived exertion (RPE),[16] as shown in Figure 1.5. This scale is based on the finding that, while exercising, a person has the ability to accurately assess how hard the body is working. It is basically a judgment call and is more appropriate when used by individuals who have been exercising for a while. The untrained exerciser typically reports a higher RPE than an athlete at the same exercise heart rate.

RPE seems to correlate strongly with other workload indicators, such as ventilation, oxygen consumption, and muscle metabolism. Participants tune into the overall sensation of effort exerted by their entire body rather than one factor such as local calf or hamstring exhaustion, panting, sweating, or body temperature. When used along with heart rate monitoring, RPE is useful for the novice, who may not be aware yet of how exercise is supposed to feel.

You might begin to make mental notes to yourself during the workout hour concerning your ratings of perceived exertion. After the workout, immediately record what you felt for each phase of the workout, expressed as numbers from 0 to 10 on the form provided in Chapter 15. Begin to notice the correlation between target heart rates achieved and how ratings of perceived exertion feel.

TALK TEST

A third and less formal method for determining aerobic intensity is called the *talk test*. It is based on the premise that, while exercising, the participant always should be able to hold a conversation. If the participant can gasp out only one or two words at a time, the exercise intensity probably is anaerobic and should be adjusted to allow for two- to three-word phrases. Because the accuracy of the talk test varies within any given population, it is best utilized in conjunction with the THR and the RPE for monitoring exercise intensity.[17]

FIGURE 1.5   Borg Scale Ratings of Perceived Exertion

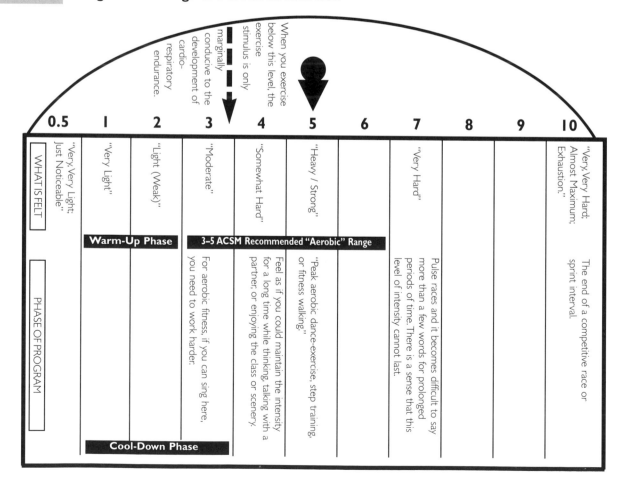

Which Method Is Best?

The experts do not agree when it comes to THR versus RPE. Some claim that only THR methods are accurate. Others believe that RPE and the talk test are more practical. Because all the methods are useful and none is consistently ideal, a good solution is to *use a combination of all three.* Once a participant has developed a good understanding of the heart rate/RPE relationship, heart rate can be monitored less frequently and RPE can be used as a primary means of measuring exercise intensity, with the talk test as an informal supplemental backup measure.[18]

Intensity Highpoints

The duration of an exercise session (20–60 minutes for cardiovascular fitness goals) is a variable element determined by the *intensity* and *impact* of your movement. (Impact is discussed fully in Chapter 7.) Once you have established your safe exercise zone, *intensity* is an easy choice to make; it is reflected by heartbeats per minute and is the result of using *the*

upper or lower end of your training zone (Figure 1.4). It is one of the small choices you must make personally and continually during each workout, according to:

- what phase of the workout you're in, and/or
- any limitations (illness, injury, etc.) to your program.

Intensity is experienced directly as the beats per minute (BPM) you count; or it is the RPE "feeling sense" of 3, 4, or 5, which quantifies how hard *you feel* you're working. Working at heart rates beyond your established safe THR zone, or an RPE of 6–7+, will result in heart rates beyond your safe zone of intensity to use during endurance exercise.

Therefore, it is helpful to monitor the intensity you're using at least twice during the aerobic segment of each workout session, by taking your pulse or quantifying your RPE. These numbers can be recorded at the conclusion of each class session, on the Fitness Journal in Chapter 15.

Goal Setting Challenge

You always have a choice. Fitness is a choice, as is understanding how to apply what you learn. With these beliefs in mind:

 Review each heading presented in Chapter 1. What question(s) come to mind regarding the information contained under those headings? Write down each point in question, on the space provided below.

_____

_____

_____

 Set an "assertiveness goal" for yourself to ask the instructor to more fully explain the above concept(s) at your next class meeting and to provide other recommended resources to read that will help clarify the point(s) you do not understand. This will facilitate your taking ownership for your learning.

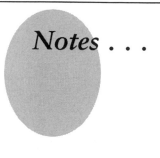

Notes . . .

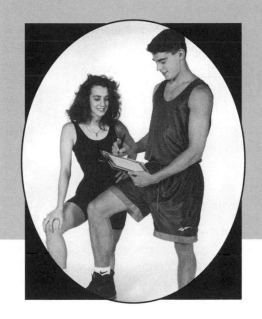

Motivation and Goal Setting

Finding the courage to change is no more difficult than learning to make one small choice at a time.

Choices, Shad Helmstetter

Taking risks and embarking on something new requires courage. Changing physical fitness status is one such situation. To be open to identifying your medical history to yourself and others takes courage. To take the risk of receiving pretesting results you don't really want to know (because you have a feeling they are not what you're going to want to hear) takes courage. And to be open to suggestions on how to significantly change a lifestyle that has become quite comfortable takes a significant act of courage.

If you have enrolled in a fitness course, celebrate the decision you have made — that first, small choice. You're on your way! The first step is behind you. If you approach becoming fit with an "eating-the-elephant-one-bite-at-a-time" mindset, each choice (each "bite") will be digested easily and become a part of you. This proactive, planned approach combined with consistent practice will become a lifestyle change that lasts.

Individuals who have a quick-fix, get-fit/lose-fat-in-a-few-weeks, reactionary mindset and a need for instant results usually become impatient with their progress. They will do too much too soon, incur injuries, or lower their resistance and physically "choke" on the big bite they're trying to take all at once.

Which is your mindset? If it is the latter, reframing it (thinking about it differently) as a methodical, proactive approach provides you with the opportunity to experience lasting results. Successes come continually when change is a one-small-choice-at-a-time process instead of one-big-end result. Celebrate your decision to change, and feel good about this one small choice. Then have patience with yourself, stay open-minded to ideas that are presented for you to consider, and enjoy the *process* of change that is now about to happen within you.

MOVING OUT OF YOUR COMFORT ZONE

Define to yourself: What are the reasons that have moved me out of my comfort zone and motivated me to take that first step, that one small choice, toward fitness? This is done internally by forming a *visual* picture in your head, listening to what you're *saying* to yourself, or connecting with how you *feel* about your physical fitness status. Do you see/taste/smell/hear/feel (experience somehow) that you:

— can't keep up and are out-of-breath while trying to accomplish everyday physical tasks?

— choose to look better cosmetically and be more attractive to yourself and others?

— have a physical ailment that you know is present because you haven't taken care of yourself?

— now choose to be the best physical specimen of a human being you can possibly become?

Write down the reasons that you pictured specifically or heard yourself say or felt within yourself. These sensory descriptions are the pleasure-seeking or pain-avoiding reasons that are motivating you. The goals you set will require you to choose methods to gain these pleasures or to avoid these pains.

MOTIVATION

True motivation lies internally within each of us. Once you identify the pleasure you're seeking or pain you're avoiding, you can elicit assistance externally, from other people or your environment, to temporarily coach and support your decision. Instructors, classmates, best friends, and attractive workout settings can give you the immediate information, encouragement, and gratification you need to get started on your fitness journey.

No one can be with you for all 1440 minutes available to you in your day to make the choices that reflect upon your fitness. Therefore, other people and your environment can be only temporary motivators in your lifetime fitness journey, because they are all external to you. It's the "kleenex analogy."[1] Use them when you need to, and then discard them and carry on!

True motivation and lasting change have to be developed or happen internally. This type of motivation is not difficult to acquire. Your internal coach is there just waiting to be called upon.[2] Internal motivation is simply a matter of understanding *how* to use your vast internal resources.

What Are My Internal Resources?

You can use your internal resources to empower you when you need motivation or to give you ideas on how to or how not to set your physical fitness goals.

Defining what these resources are within you will give you the key to accessing and enhancing your future and provide you with the ability to set powerful goals. These resources consist of:

- hereditary and environmental influences to date
- positive and negative life experiences
- wants, needs, priorities, and goals
- strengths, talents, and interests
- weaknesses, risk factors, and poor choices
- beliefs/truths/rules you follow
- attitudes (interpreting an experience as positive or negative)
- feelings (emotions)
- actions/behaviors/choices you've expressed (resulting from all of the above)

Take a contemplative moment and review these points. What mental pictures, self-talk, and feelings surface as thoughts reflecting your life experiences, needs, wants, and goals? In terms of your physical fitness, the resources that surface will represent pleasureful or painful memories — thoughts and resulting actions that you'll choose to experience again and ones you don't choose to experience ever again!

Moving toward pleasureful results and away from painful ones are the forces behind motivation. The direction you've just stated (toward pleasure or away from pain) reflects how you've stored your internal resources.

> *Your internal resources are thoughts reflecting*
> *— past and present life experiences*
> *— past, present, and future needs, wants, and goals.[3]*

How Internal Resources Affect Motivation

The point to understand with motivation is how you have stored your thoughts (internal resources) sensory-wise regarding your physical fitness. Do you remember an earlier attempt at aerobics, step training, fitness walking, strength training, or stretching as a positive experience that met your goal at the time? How do you picture, hear, taste, smell, self-talk, and feel about that experience? You might say, "Great workout! I was energized and made lots friends!" or, "The room smelled terrible. I'll never go back there!"

What answers your thoughts are your *sensory representations.* Visual pictures, sounds, tastes, or smells come to mind. You can hear yourself stating the two examples just given. A feeling comes over you that is either pleasant or painful. Motivation has the following sensory components:

1. Images, sounds, tastes, smells.
2. Internal self-talk.
3. Body sensations (movements, touch, emotions).

IMAGES, SOUNDS, TASTES, SMELLS

Individuals should take ownership of (responsibility for) how they are picturing or imaging the fitness goals they're choosing to set. Images that are big, bright, in color, and moving are more powerful than small, dim, black and white, freeze-frame images. The same applies to tastes, sounds, and smells. They are fresh or tangy, soft or loud, strong or weak. Ask yourself, "How *large* are the images I'm making in my head? Are they small like a postcard or large as a poster?" More powerful images are more motivating. Goals established with powerful images will be accomplished much more quickly.

SELF-TALK

Internal dialogue that is in the present tense, positive, and enabling is more motivating than self-talk that is in the past tense or future tense, negative, and disabling. For example, "I am confident of my ability to learn new aerobics moves quickly and am enjoying my instructor's creative, improvising style" is more powerfully motivating than stating to oneself, "I will feel confident of my ability in aerobics class as soon as I learn all the basic moves and get to know the instructor." Listen to the verbs and adverbs in your sentences, and construct talk that is *as if it's already accomplished*. An assessment of your Self-Talk is provided in Chapter 15.

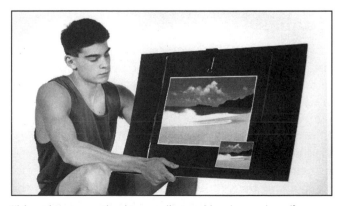

"How large are the images I'm making in my head? Are they small like a postcard or large as a poster?"

BODY SENSATIONS

Body sensations that focus on gaining pleasure instead of avoiding pain ("doing my best" instead of "not coming in last") and sensations that are quick, powerful, big, high, and the like are the most motivating. For example, if you want to get up in the morning and are lying in the comfort of bed, what will motivate you to get up? Actually, what *did* motivate you to get up at 6:30 a.m. on a Saturday morning this past winter? Did you:

- picture how cold, gray, and dreary it was outside,
- say, "Gosh, it's so *early*, and I'm so *tired*,"

and slowly move out of bed?

or did you:

- picture, taste, smell a fun event you had planned for the day,
- say to yourself, "It's great to be alive! Today is a fresh new day with no mistakes,"

and spring up quickly?

If you're not motivated to do something you must change your images, tastes, sounds, smells, self-talk, movements, touch, and feelings.

Changing Sensory Representations

According to established research on eye and head positions during various modes of thought,[4, 5, 6, 7] when you are making *visual pictures*, your head is at chin level or higher (Figure 2.1). Your eyes are looking forward or up, and to one side or the other. In the *remembered* pictures, the eyes are up and to one side of you or up and forward. In the *constructed* pictures made as when *goal setting* (future pictures), can't recall, or recall incorrectly, the eyes are up and to the other side (the opposite side from the remembered images) or up and forward.

When remembering or constructing *sounds and words*, the eyes turn toward the ears in a horizontal movement. The *remembered* sounds/words are accessed toward the memory side. The sounds/words not experienced yet, can't recall, or recall incorrectly, are accessed toward the *constructed* side.

When carrying on *internal dialogue* (engaging in positive or negative self-talk), the head will lower, the chin will drop, you will be looking down and to one side, and talking to yourself (Figure 2.2). When

FIGURE 2.1

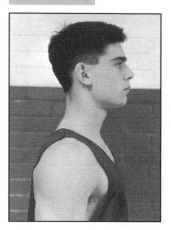

Accessing visual images.

FIGURE 2.2

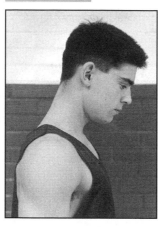

Accessing self-talk or feelings, touch, movement.

you access how you *feel*, especially painful emotions such as anger, sadness, and fear, you again will be in the lowered head and chin position, looking down and to the other side (opposite the self-talk side).

The *location sides* of memory, self-talk, constructed thought, and feelings are individual. They can be determined easily by you or by others observing you. Directional movement of your hand gestures, predicates in your sentences, and physiologies in addition to the eye movement further clarify how you store and retrieve information.

The "eye accessing" information may be new to you. It can be a *key* element to understanding your internal resources and what motivates you. It can assist you with setting and achieving powerful goals, which may have eluded you in the past. Once you understand how you make images, sounds, smells, taste, self-talk, and the body sensations of movement, touch, and feelings, you will know exactly how and where to begin the change process.

Another excellent example may clarify accessing and how you've stored your thoughts. Picture in your mind experiencing first "the thrill of victory" and then "the agony of defeat." When people are experiencing *victory*, physiologically the head and chin are level or up. When they are experiencing *defeat*, physiologically the head and chin lower, and feelings or self-talk are tapped into while in the chin-down position. To get out of this agony-of-defeat mindset, you literally must keep your chin up so you no longer are accessing the disabling feelings or self-talk spatially located down.

Any change or goal setting must begin at the sensory representation, internal-thought level.

KEEPING THE POWER TO CHANGE

To use your full potential to set powerful goals, you must take ownership of your internal resources. This requires you to take responsibility and not blame others or the environment for your successes and failures. When you retain ownership of your physical fitness program goals, this provides you with the ability to change, to set powerful goals that *you* choose, and to go about the business of systematically achieving them.

If a goal you're setting for yourself doesn't happen soon enough, and any type of blame enters the internal picturing, feelings, and self-talk, stop. Take ownership and state. "*I own this situation. How can I get the results I need? How can I repicture or talk differently about this situation so it is helpful to me?*" Taking ownership of your internal resources — your thoughts — is the key to personal freedom and to all goal achievement. You have a free will and are in charge of your life. Enjoy the freedom and choose wisely, one small choice at a time!

GOAL-SETTING STRATEGIES

It's time to apply your new knowledge of internal motivation and plan your future by first acknowledging, and perhaps reestablishing, your priorities, in order to set powerful goals.

Establishing Priorities

Priorities refer to how you spend your time, and are the means to reach your goals (the ends you seek). Figure 2.3 can be used to set your top 20 priorities. It allows you to identify how many hours per day and week you devote to each priority, and to record time robbers that take you away from a priority. Can you identify an excellent role model whom you associate with each? Role models provide us time-saving, short-cut ideas on how to do something the quickest, most efficient, and best way possible. Take advantage of their strategies whenever possible by asking them *how* they do what they do.

FIGURE 2.3 **Establishing Priorities**

Priorities are the means to your ends. They are things you give time to in the wellness areas of your physical / social / emotional / spiritual / intellectual / talent expression dimensions.

Top 20 Priorities (Listed In Any Order)	Hours Each Day	Hours Each Week	Time Robbers	Role Model	Rank Order of Importance
•					#
•					#
•					#
•					#
•					#
•					#
•					#
•					#
•					#
•					#
•					#
•					#
•					#
•					#
•					#
•					#
•					#
•					#
•					#
•					#

In the last column of the figure, you can rank each priority by how you now feel about it (not which takes the most time). The key to setting powerful goals is to be certain that your time has been prioritized to include these goals, to enable them to happen.

Creating The Future in Advance

The foundation for successful goal setting has been established:

1. Identifying *reasons* you're choosing to change
2. Becoming aware of how you're motivated — which senses are used and how — and, consequently, how to change your actions at the sensory-thought level
3. Assessing and reestablishing your time priorities, to enable change to happen.

The goal-setting procedure tells your brain precisely what goal you are choosing to set. It provides solid reasoning for why you're etching this goal-set groove. It also breaks old programming by presenting your pain-avoidance reasons. Positive action

choices are made immediately to create the motivational pictures, self-talk, and movements necessary to initiate active change in your exercise program. Making an audiotape of yourself responding to the statements and questions for each goal you set may prove helpful. You'll find that the repetition of this blueprinting process is a unique short-cut to achieving your goals. During the goal-setting process, one end to keep in mind always is to have *fun* during your pursuit of fitness!

Setting goals helps to keep you focused on daily improvement and positive change. It encourages consistency in your fitness program and helps to keep you on target. Without goals, there's nothing to shoot for!

When they are properly set internally and nourished continually, goals will become reality. Believe it, and you will see it. Your future resides within you as a rich resource of possibilities.

> *One simple decision:*
> *consciously*
> *actively*
> *make your choices.*
>
> *Choices*, Shad Helmstetter

Developing Goal Scripts for Chapter 2

For each goal you set, both now and at the end of every chapter, consider the following four statements and questions. Using one or several full sentences for each section, write down your immediate responses. All of the responses to these four segments of a goal, collectively, become one "goal script" — the precise language you'll repeat to yourself twice daily until you achieve the goal.

1 State one goal in positive, *present-tense* language. Ask yourself, "What will I experience — see, hear, taste, smell, feel — when I achieve it? You'll recognize these as the components of motivation. All powerful goals use the SMART formula: specific, measurable, achievable, realistic, timely.

_____

_____

2 State your *pleasure-value reasons*. Ask yourself, "Why am I totally committed to achieving each goal?" Involve your values to answer this question. Values may be any of the following: adventure and change, commitment, freedom, giving pleasure to others, happiness, health, love, power, prestige and worth, security, life purpose, success, expression of talent, trust, loyalty, and any other values important to you.

_____

_____

3 State your *pain-avoidance value reasons*. Because we do more to avoid pain than to gain pleasure, heap on the painful thoughts so you're really motivated to change! Break the link of the old programmed ways by asking yourself, "What painful values do I choose to avoid?" Some pain-avoidance values are: anger or resentment, anxiety or worry, boredom, depression, embarrassment, frustration, guilt, humiliation, jealousy, feeling overwhelmed, physical pain, prejudice, rejection, sadness.

_____

_____

4 Reestablish the pleasure link by picturing, hearing, feeling, "What *actions* do I choose to take or do immediately to master this goal? What is something I can start doing right now and within the next 24 hours?"

_____

_____

Safety First

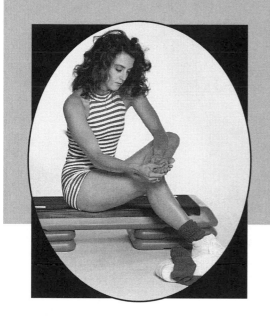

All physical activities have an element of risk. By taking proper preventive measures, however, problems and injuries can be minimized. The following discussion will alert you to some of the more common concerns.

Self-discipline is required to become and stay physically fit. The dividends of wellness and vitality are well worth it. Some general tips for sensible training are:

1. Progress gradually in your sessions.

2. Be sure to both warm up and cool down.

3. Progress from easy to advanced in the stretches, aerobic options, and strength-training exercises.

4. Do not perform to the point of exhaustion. Learn to read your body signs. You're going to perspire, and you're going to tire a little. With an effective fitness program, you may encounter some initial, slight, temporary discomfort.

5. Pace yourself. For example, after engaging in numerous aerobics moves, a complete step-training routine, or one lap in your fitness walking, you may be short of breath. This should subside within minutes. If it doesn't, you've worked too hard.

6. If you are unsure about a specific discomfort or pain, ask a reliable person (i.e., your physician) about it before continuing with activity.

SIGNS OF OVEREXERTION

Monitoring your pulse helps determine how hard to exercise your body, but you also need to be aware of your own bodily signs of overexertion. Signs are:

- Severe breathlessness.

- Poor heart rate response (continually monitoring too high an exercising heart rate that does not drop significantly after 1 minute of recovery, or final heart rate not below 120 beats per minute after 5 minutes of cool-down.

- Undue fatigue during exercise and inability to recover from a workout later in the day.

- Insomnia.

- Persistent, severe muscle soreness. (The type of muscle soreness to guard against is not immediate but becomes apparent 24–48 hours after exercise.)

- Nausea, feeling faint, dizziness.

- Tightness or pains in the chest.

These symptoms do not indicate that you shouldn't exercise. Rather, they suggest a reduced level of activity until you develop the capacity to handle more intense workouts. An exercise program should be undertaken cautiously, and the frequency, intensity and duration of each session increased gradually.

An exercise program should be undertaken cautiously, and the frequency, intensity, and duration of each session increased gradually.

If you have any of the following symptoms, ease gradually to a slow walk, sit with your head between your knees, or lie down on your back and elevate your feet. The latter will help the blood move to your head more readily and carry the needed oxygen to your brain. If any of these symptoms persist, contact your doctor.

1. Abnormal heart action

   - Irregular pulse.
   - Fluttering, jumping, or palpitations in chest or throat.
   - Sudden burst of rapid heartbeats.
   - Sudden, very slow pulse when a moment before it had been on target (immediate or delayed).

2. Pain or pressure in the center of the chest or the arm or throat precipitated by exercise or following exercise (immediate or delayed).

3. Dizziness, lightheadedness, sudden incoordination, confusion, cold sweat, glassy stare, pallor, blueness, or fainting (immediate).

   Do not try to cool down. Stop exercise and lie down with your feet elevated, or put your head down between your legs until the symptoms pass.[1]

SAFETY VARIABLES

Numerous variables can affect a fitness program. These include presence of illness, infection, or injury, lack of exercise for a while, location and environment, and shoe selection, among others.

Presence of Illness, Infection, or Injury

Illness, infection, or injury will show up in your "thermometer of fitness," your pulse. It will be higher at rest and will escalate to the training zone with less than your usual effort. In that event, take it easy and decide whether to "walk" through your program mentally to maintain your discipline of exercising or to curtail exercise until you're completely well again.

Missing a While?

If you have missed aerobic exercise for a time, return to it slowly. When you miss activity several times, you will need to start more cautiously, as if beginning a new program. For example, you may have a bout of flu and are unable to exercise for a week. When you are able to exercise again, do not plan to start where you left off. Return cautiously to the fitness level you were at before the illness.

A leading cardiologist in the United States has stated that you will lose approximately half of your fitness program gains after just 5 weeks if you discontinue your program totally. After 10 weeks of no aerobic activity, you will have lost most of your fitness gains.[2] Whenever a circumstance curtails your program, return to it slowly and systematically.

Location and Environment

Select a convenient and physiologically safe location for your workouts. Choose a *wood*-based floor or an area carpeted with flat nap and thick padding. (Carpeted surfaces tend to make lateral moves and turns risky, however.) Try not to exercise on concrete, as it has no "give" or buoyancy. Concrete surfaces impose unnecessary stress on your legs and feet.

   A resilient floor should be selected for exercise that involves repeated foot impacts. If such a surface is not available, the exercise routines should be modified to ensure that the feet remain close to the floor throughout the program (low-impact exercises).[3]

If relative humidity is high and the temperature is 85° (room or outside), curtail your aerobics, step training, or fitness walking program. Seek another option, such as aerobic swimming in a cool-air environment.

For aerobic exercise a cold environment is fine as long as you protect yourself thoroughly, especially your air passages. (At 40° F. and below cover your air passages.) Heat, however, does matter. Heat stress injuries can occur if caution is abandoned.

SHOE SELECTION

The shoes you wear constitute one of your major requirements. When you jump or run, you place three to six times more force on your feet than when you are stationary. If you weigh 125 pounds, you are placing 375 to 750 pounds of pressure on your feet with each jump. Your body can withstand the stress of exercise better if you wear shoes that shock-absorb this pressure or exercise on a surface with a giving quality. Select a shoe that totally supports your foot for your exercise modality. The following criteria and Table 3.1[4] give specific guidelines for personalizing your shoe selection.

- Inquire about midsole composition. For durability and performance, select shoes made from either compression-molded ethyl vinyl acetate (EVA) or polyurethane.

- Stay with the same brand and model of shoe you are replacing if it has been satisfactory.

- Do not allow yourself to be forced or pressured into buying a shoe that does not feel comfortable.

- About every 4 months replace a single pair of shoes worn at least 4 days per week for any fitness-related activity. If the shoes have a polyurethane midsole, the wear may be extended up to 6 months. If they have a standard, open-cell EVA midsole, they may last only 3 months.

- Examine the inside of the shoe as well as the insole. Shoes with removable insoles are preferable because they tend to be better cushioned and allow the fit of a custom foot orthotic, if needed.[5]

- Get nylon uppers rather than leather uppers if you want a cooler shoe. If you prefer an all-leather shoe, be sure it has ventilation holes on the top and sides. Extra design leather or suede along the ball edge of the foot area (toes) provides longer shoe life.

- Choose a shoe that has a sole with a relatively smooth tread[6] and of white rubber, designed for aerobics or court use (Figure 3.1). Jogging shoes with black rubber soles, designed for road and track running and with rubber triangles,

TABLE 3.1	Personalizing Your Shoe Selection
IF YOU:	**PICK A SHOE THAT:**
are heavier or taller	has a firm, dense midsole, like polyurethane (PU).
are lighter or smaller	has a softer midsole, like compression-molded ethyl vinyl acetate (EVA).
have a high arch	is well-cushioned and soft.
have a flexible arch or flat foot	is firm and has motion-control features.
IF YOU HAVE HAD:	**PICK A SHOE THAT:**
stress fractures	is cushioned in the midsole and insole.
plantar fasciitis	is flexible and has a well-contoured insole with a prominent arch support.
ankle sprains	has a firm PU midsole with a ¾"-high reinforced upper.
shin splints	has an elevated heel, plenty of cushion, and a contoured arch insole.
knee problems	has a firm sole with lateral reinforcement in the upper.
IF YOU PARTICIPATE IN:	**YOU NEED:**
aerobics/dance-exercise only	an aerobic dance shoe or a cross trainer. If you have had arch or heel problems, choose an aerobics shoe because it is more flexible.
weight training, stair climbing* and stationary biking	a cross trainer.
aerobics/dance-exercise, weight training, stair climbing and biking	a cross trainer or aerobics shoe with a PU midsole.
aerobics/dance-exercise and running	an aerobics shoe and a running shoe.
aerobics/dance-exercise and fitness walking	an aerobics shoe and either a walking shoe or a running shoe.

*Step training is included here.

From "How to Choose Shoes," by Douglas H. Richie, *IDEA Today*, April 1991, p. 67.

FIGURE 3.1

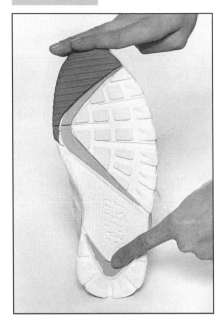

A sole with the rubber designed for sideward movement, and the heel unflaired.

FIGURE 3.2   **FIGURE 3.3**

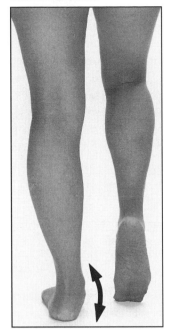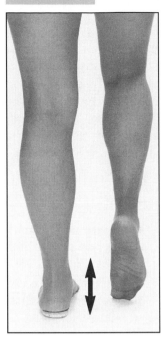

Pronation.   Correction with a sports orthotic.[8]

squares, circles, or thick waves provide excellent forward movement, but because aerobics consists of forward, backward, and lateral movement, this is not the best choice of shoe sole.

> The rough treads of most running shoes can be hazardous during aerobic exercise dance as they can cause the feet to come to an abrupt halt each time they strike the floor. Thus, most shoes designed for running are unsuitable for aerobic dance.[7]

- If you have a tendency toward *pronated ankles* (lower leg bones do not sit directly on the ankle, as shown in Figure 3.2) do not select a wide heel flair of rubber. This heel flair will limit, to some extent, your lateral (sideward) movement and also will not provide the appropriate correction to avoid possible future injury to naturally weak ankles, as it does in jogging, which is all forward movement. Pronation of ankles can be corrected inside the shoe by means of:
  - an extra firm heel box.
  - raising the arch with a specifically designed wedge.
  - controlling the floor contact of various portions of the foot by a specially designed orthotic (prescribed corrective device) for the foot, as shown in Figure 3.3.

Sports orthotics are devices that are custom-made to control the function of your unique foot specifically. They are not arch supports. Requiring several weeks of construction, they are shaped to *control your foot closely the entire time it is on the floor or ground*. The bones in your foot are moved so the muscles can function and adapt normally, decreasing or eliminating foot problems. The orthotics are made of an unbreakable, reinforced material and are worn inside your athletic shoe.[8]

A person doesn't have to live with the pain that structural imbalances cause, such as aching on the entire bottom of the foot from the forward movement of running or shin splints from the lateral movement of aerobics. Sports orthotics can be prescribed by a qualified specialist, such as a podiatrist.

PROPER CLOTHING

Choosing what to wear for the environment in which you are exercising is important. Safety, comfort, and ease of movement are the variables for aerobics apparel. It is best to dress in layers. A warm-up sweatsuit or jogging suit will help increase the temperature of your arm and leg muscles during warm-up. On very warm or highly humid and warm days this, of course, is unnecessary. Cotton material is best, as it absorbs perspiration better than other fabrics. When cotton clothing becomes damp, the surrounding air causes the moisture to evaporate, and this cools the body.

During laps or routines you'll need to be free to move in all directions and sweat freely. Therefore, choose to wear as little as possible, especially when the temperature and relative humidity are high. Long, loose slacks should be avoided, as they can catch under the feet. The same is true for tight-fitting garments, as they restrict flexibility. The best advice for someone who exercises vigorously is to keep clothing to a comfortable minimum. This allows unrestricted motion and facilitates loss of excessive body heat.[9]

Exercise apparel kept to a comfortable minimum is a solid guideline for all participants, to avoid heat stress injuries. Individuals who are overweight or obese are prime targets for overheating because they have a thick layer of fat tissue between internal organs and the outside layer of skin. It works like insulation and keeps in internal heat. The internal body systems may overheat and cause heat exhaustion or heat stroke. Therefore, don't try to "sweat" off water pounds by wearing lots of clothing or rubber-lined sweatsuits. Sweat and water loss are bodily cooling mechanisms and are not to be used as a measurement for weight loss. Water is *not* fat!

To prevent friction in your shoes, wear cotton socks without wrinkles. Cotton absorbs sweat. This will help to keep your feet drier and free from blisters.

Finally, wearing a towel around the neck during exercise is contrary to all physiological principles. The major artery from the heart to the brain is located in the neck area, and it has to be free for cooling by exposure to air of the skin surface in that area.

FLUID INTAKE

Water is the principal means of transporting heat (and substances) within the body. In warm environments (meaning within a room or a geographical setting), it is the *only* means of dispersing body heat. This is accomplished by the evaporation of released perspiration on the surface of the skin. When the room air contacts the sweat, the skin surface is cooled, and the cooling then is conducted internally. Production of body heat increases greatly during physical exercise.

Unless water for perspiration is available, the body temperature increases beyond normal, causing overheating. When fluid loss exceeds supply, dehydration follows. When dehydration sets in, even modest physical activity causes the heart rate and body temperature to increase. When the water loss is approximately 5% of the total body water, evidence of heat exhaustion may become apparent. When losses are 10%, the condition may lead to heat stroke soon. This is fatal unless the person receives immediate attention (through submersion in an ice bath).

As the work level and environmental temperature increase, fluid intake must be increased to maintain fluid balance.[10] Because there is no basis for restricting water intake during aerobics and no evidence that humans can adapt or be trained to tolerate water intake lower than daily losses, you should replace water loss by continuous daily fluid intake. A few guidelines to facilitate water balance are as follows.

1. Drink plenty of liquids at least 20 minutes before beginning an aerobic exercise hour. Frequent, small intake of fluid throughout the day is best.

2. If you have been drinking plenty of water prior to aerobic sessions, you probably will not need to drink water during the session (room temperature and humidity usually are the determining variables). If you get thirsty, however, drink water. Your thirst mechanism is a late sign that you need water, so don't ignore it.

3. After aerobic exercise, relax and sit with a tall glass of ice water or an inexpensive, homemade electrolyte ("sports drink") solution:[11]

   1 qt. frozen reconstituted orange juice
   3 qts. water
   ½ tsp. salt

   This will provide immediate rehydration and is a pleasant way to conclude your session.

4. If you use any of the sports beverages or commercial preparations, dilute them with water to decrease the concentration of sugar and thus decrease the time the fluid stays in the stomach. Recommended dilutions are given in Table 3.2.[12] Many "sports beverages" are promoted as sources of available sodium, potassium, and sugar. Replacement needs for sodium and potassium can be met much better through a diet that contains a variety of foods and supplies these

TABLE 3.2 Dilution of Replacement Fluids

Fluid	Concentration
Fruit juices	1 part juice; 3 parts water
Soft drinks	1 part soda; 3 parts water
Vegetable juices	1 part juice; 1 part water
Gatorade®	1 part drink; 1 part water
Pripps Pluss®	1 part drink; 3 parts water
Quickick® (orange flavor)	1 part drink; 3 parts water

and other nutrients, including proper amounts of water.

Deliberate dehydration (by loading on the clothes and promoting profuse sweating), of course, is not an acceptable method of weight control. This will cause a temporary loss of weight, which is regained rapidly by rehydration. Loss of weight should be body fat, not water or protein.

COMMON INJURIES

Blisters

Blisters arise in seconds but take days to heal. Even a small blister that goes untreated will affect your workout. The best advice is to do everything you can to prevent blisters from forming in the first place.

Blisters are caused by friction as the surface of the shoe rubs against the skin of the foot. Wear shoes that fit well. They should not be too loose or too tight. To help prevent blisters, lubricate the trouble spot with petroleum jelly before you put on your shoes for a fitness session. If you sweat a lot, powder your feet also. Because improperly fitting shoes are the culprit, be sure to do a few exertive moves in your local shoe store to size up comfort *in motion* before purchasing the shoes.

If you get a water blister, care for it as follows:

- Scrub the area gently with soap and water to thoroughly clean it.
- Gently swab with alcohol or a surgical preparation.
- Make two incisions at the outer edges of the blister. Slowly press out the superficial fluid.
- Apply ointment or first-aid cream.
- Bandage until healed completely.

If you get a blood blister, care for it as follows:

- Ice the area.
- Do not puncture. The chance of infection is great, as it connects with the circulatory system.
- Place a "doughnut"-type compress around the blister until it is reabsorbed and healed completely.

Bunions

A bunion is a large, bony protuberance on the outside of the big toe that indicates joint inflammation. The main causes of bunions are overpronation and faulty foot structure. A podiatrist is the specialist to see to correct bunions.

Muscle Cramps

A cramp is a painful muscle spasm. Cramping may occur during or following a vigorous exercise session. It is the result of two different phenomena. Muscle cramping *during* an exercise session usually reflects an electrolyte and fluid imbalance in your system.[13] Electrolytes are sodium, calcium, chloride, potassium, and magnesium. Cramping usually occurs because you have not properly replaced your water loss while conditioning and training.

If a person has lost a lot of water through perspiration (8 or more pounds of water), those elements have to be replaced. With moderate sweating and water loss, regular, daily water intake and proper diet will replace the needed fluids and electrolytes and do much to eliminate this type of cramping.

The most common cramps associated with exercise are those occurring in the *24* hours *after* exercise, especially after having gone to bed or after a sudden movement. These cramps (post-exercise) are not associated with electrolyte imbalance.[14] They are believed to be caused by swelling of muscle fiber, agitating the peripheral nerves that service the muscle tissue. If these cramps are frequent and severe, the treatment prescribed may be .2 grams of quinine sulfate.

Immediate relief for cramping is to do a static stretch in the exact opposite direction for a few moments.

Muscle Soreness

Two types of pain are associated with severe muscular exercise:

1. Pain during and immediately after exercise, which may persist for several hours.
2. Localized soreness that usually does not appear for 24 to 48 hours.

The first is associated with metabolic wastes on pain receptors and the second with torn muscle fibers or connective tissue.[15] The first type need not cause great concern; it presents no lasting problems. The delayed type requires attention in the form of a more adequate warm-up and cool-down stretching program and the incorporation of a strength segment into your program. Gradual, sensible muscle use during exercise is the best prevention.

Muscle, Tendon, and Joint Injuries

For *muscle strains or sprains*, the treatment is to ICE (ice, compress, and elevate). Injuries are iced (or cold whirlpools are administered) to inhibit swelling and promote healing by making the body internally (rather than at the surface) supply more blood to the affected deep-problem area. The body forces more blood to come to the area when cold applications are applied by making the body work harder pumping away the old cells and pumping in fresh oxygen and nutrients to begin the repair process at the deep site rather than at the surface skin area.

Ice applications are administered two times a day, about 20 minutes each time. When the affected area no longer is warm to the touch (using the back of your hand) but seems to be the same temperature as the surrounding area, ice compresses can be stopped.

When heat is applied, it brings an increase of blood to the skin surface, but it doesn't make the body work hard at all on its own to pump in a fresh supply of oxygen and nutrients to the deep affected area. The less comfortable application of ice will hasten the repair process.

Achilles tendonitis is an inflammation of the thick tendon that connects the heel to the calf muscle. This injury results from wearing shoes with inadequately thick soles that do not provide a proper cushion for the foot. Aggravating the problem are biomechanical problems such as bowed legs, tight hamstrings and calves, high-arched feet, over-pronation, and excessive toe-running.

Adequate heel-cord stretching helps prevent Achilles tendonitis. Any aggravation of this problem can cause a serious and permanent condition; anyone experiencing this problem should not continue to exercise with the pain.

Shin Splints

The most common injury to new aerobics enthusiasts is shin splints, characterized by pain on the front and inside of the lower leg (Figure 3.4). Although it is common in runners, this malady can affect anyone who engages in physical activity using the legs. Most cases of shin splints occur at the *beginning* of an exercise program because the lower leg muscles are weak.

Jumping and running activities cause the leg muscles in the back of the leg to develop and become stronger while the leg muscles in front develop only slightly. This muscle imbalance can cause shin splints if it is not treated correctly.[16] When the strength of one muscle or muscle group is disproportionate to that of the antagonist(s) for that muscle or group, the weaker muscle should be strengthened to restore balance around the joint.[17]

Preventive measures include light, flexible shoes with good arch support. Track running should be avoided as the repeated turns put great stress on the lower leg. Stretching before and after physical activity helps the muscles absorb shock. Performing a stretch using three repetitions of straight-leg and bent-knee wall leans for 20 seconds may alleviate

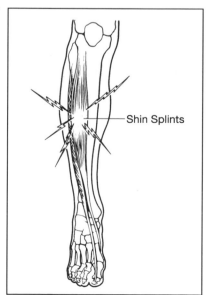

Shin splints.

the problem (Figure 3.5). Another preventive measure is to develop the strength of the anterior lower leg area. This can be accomplished by performing an exercise such as the lower-leg flexor, using a towel rolled lengthwise or resistance/rubber tubing. Sit tall with your legs together in front of you and place the center of the towel or tubing securely under the toes of your shoes. Place your hands comfortably in front of the abdomen and don't move them during the exercise. Slowly point your toes down and toward the wall in front of you (Figure 3.6) and hold 15 seconds. Relax a few seconds, then flex your feet at the ankle and draw your toes up tightly toward your knees (Figure 3.7) and hold 15 seconds. Repeat the entire exercise for several minutes. This can be done one leg at a time or both feet working together simultaneously.

Of utmost importance in caring for shin splints are *rest and immediate icing* in the tender area. The icing should be for 8–10 continuous minutes while gently massaging the problem area. Later in the day a second gentle ice massage for the same time duration should be done to give the desired relief. This procedure should be followed for several days. You'll be amazed how quickly you will heal within one week.

FIGURE 3.5

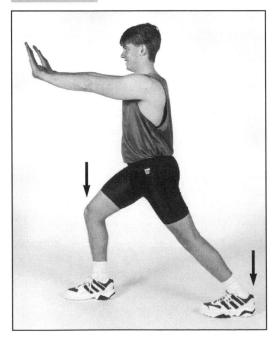

Exercise for relief of shin splints.

FIGURE 3.6

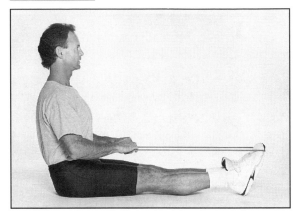

Strength exercise to develop the anterior lower leg muscles, **down** position.

FIGURE 3.7

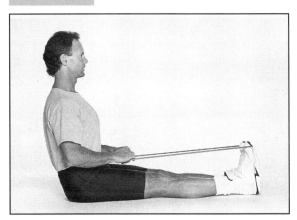

Strength exercise to develop the anterior lower leg muscles, **up** position.

If icing, rest, aspirin (four to six per day), strengthening, and stretching do not create relief within 10 days, see a physician to rule out more serious conditions such as stress fractures, structural imbalances that might require orthotics, or anterior compartment syndrome.[18]

DRUG USE

As many as half of all deaths from heart attack may occur because of "electrical failure," not "pump failure," of the heart. People with adequate heart muscles die because their heart's electrical signals get out of sync; the muscle then twitches chaotically and no longer can pump blood. Known as *ventricular fibrillation*, this rhythm disturbance is deadly if it cannot be reversed within minutes.[19] In recent years the drug-related deaths of superstar athletes by cocaine intoxication are related directly to this phenomenon.

PROFESSIONAL HELP

Understanding cause and effect will help prevent problems or injuries during the quest for fitness. Whenever problems or injuries do arise, you should seek out answers from qualified professionals — medical doctors, sports medicine specialists, physiologists, athletic trainers.

Follow the diet, exercise, and mental training programs promoted by scientific professionals. Read and believe authors whose credentials are impressive in the various fields of total fitness and who publish their researched findings in professional journals. In this way, you will have access to the most accurate, up-to-date knowledge available, and a more safe, fun way to good health.

Goal Setting Challenge

 Correct any safety concern or fear you may have that you have let slide without proper attention.

Developing Goal Scripts for Chapter 3

DIRECTIONS: Write complete sentences for each segment below. Combine your responses to all four segments. This goal script is designed around your needs and choices. Read it (or make an audiotape and play it) twice daily, morning and evening, until you master it.

1 State one goal in positive, *present-tense* language. Ask yourself, "What will I experience — see, hear, taste, smell, feel — in regard to the results? Keep in mind that all powerful goals use the SMART formula: specific, measurable, achievable, realistic, timely.

_____

_____

2 State your *pleasure-value reasons.* Ask yourself, "Why am I totally committed to achieving this goal? What am I choosing to feel?"

_____

_____

3 State your *pain-avoidance value reasons.* Ask yourself, "What painful values do I choose to avoid feeling?"

_____

_____

4 State *immediate action(s)* you can take in the next 24 hours. Use positive, present-tense verbs such as *choose* and verbs ending with "ing."

_____

_____

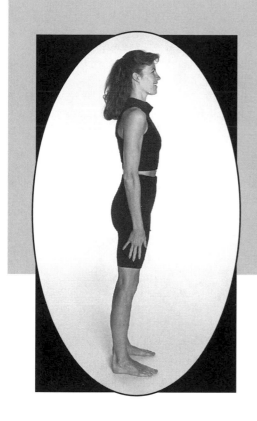

Posture and Positioning

The best reason to include posture information in a fitness course is to *save your back!* To ensure that you are exercising in the safest possible fashion, you must understand good postural techniques, regardless of the activity. Poor posture is illustrated in Figure 4.1. Correct posture is shown in Figure 4.2.

THE MECHANICS

The downward pressure of gravity applied to the bones of the upright, balanced skeleton tends to cause it to buckle at three principal points: hip, knee, and ankle. Because the body weight is largely in front of the spinal column, the body tends to fall forward. To counteract these tendencies toward buckling and falling forward, five muscles or muscle groups are antigravity in nature, allowing for an upright, balanced skeleton. The antigravity muscle groups responsible for holding us erect are located in the:

- back (along with the spinal column)
- abdomen
- buttocks
- front of the thighs
- calves.

To develop good posture, the position of the spine, pelvic girdle, and hip joints (which act as the main hinges of the body) have to be controlled. This is done primarily by the five muscle groups. *How* you control them determines posture.

FIGURE 4.1	**FIGURE 4.2**
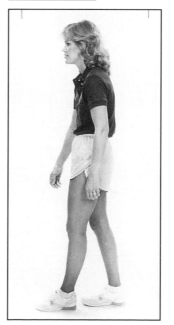	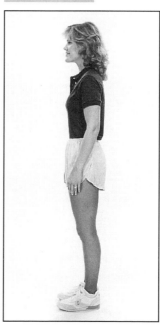
Poor posture.	Good posture.

Balanced Static Posture

A balanced standing posture is established when:

- The head and stretched neck are balanced on top of the spine and centered above the shoulders, while keeping the chin parallel to the floor.

- The shoulders are pulled back and down in a relaxed position.

- The chest and rib cage are raised up.

- The abdominal muscles are pulled in and up, under the rib cage.

- The pelvic girdle is pulled down and under, tightening the buttocks. The pelvis rests on the two thigh bones balanced over two arched feet.

- The knees are relaxed. Locking the knees in a hyperextended position causes imbalance and increases susceptibility to knee injury.

- The weight is distributed equally on both feet while standing with the feet parallel and toes pointing forward, taking the weight on the outer half of the feet.

- The arms are relaxed.

Poor Posture

If any part of the body is out of alignment, weight distribution will be uneven over the base of support and will put unnecessary strain on muscles, bones, and joints. This soon causes fatigue.

Poor posture is a habit that can be changed but it takes time, for it has been a part of a person for a long time (Figure 4.3).

Most muscles are in pairs. If a muscle is shortened constantly, its opposing muscle lengthens and becomes weak from disuse. Therefore, stretching (lengthening) one set of muscles while simultaneously contracting (shortening) the opposing set of muscles, and then repeating vice versa, will strengthen both, especially if additional weight resistance is used.

With this information, you can understand why stretching and strengthening the muscles will lead to better posture. If your body is to move freely, every muscle has to be able to shorten or lengthen in either a strong, quick manner or a slow, relaxed manner. Fully understanding the principles of stretching and strength training will assist you further in understanding and obtaining good posture goals.

FIGURE 4.3   **Characteristics of Poor Posture**

SIDE VIEWS

"Fatigue Slump"
"Debutante Slouch"

1. Head and chin are forward
2. Chest sags
3. Shoulders are forward and in
4. Abdomen sags
5. Back is inclined to the rear
6. Pelvis is pushed forward
7. Knees are locked
8. Body line zigzags

"Hollow Back"

1. Head is back and chin up
2. Chest is high
3. Shoulders are back
4. Abdomen protrudes
5. Back curves are accentuated
6. Pelvis is tilted forward (lordosis)
7. Knees are forward
8. Body line zigzags

BACK VIEW

1. Head is tilted
2. Body is asymmetrical
3. "Humpback" (kyphosis)
4. One shoulder is higher than the other
5. Spinal column curves sideward
6. One hip is high and protruding
7. Kneecap turns out or in
8. Ankles roll inward
9. Feet point outward
10. Weight is distributed unequally on feet, on inner border of foot (pronation)

Efficient Positions

If you now have poor posture during aerobic movement activities, you will have to reeducate your neuromuscular system. This takes patience, persistence, and a sincere desire to want to improve your appearance and the efficiency of your body.

If you were born free from hereditary or congenital deformities, you can obtain good posture (Figure 4.4). It's all a matter of:

- understanding balanced postures.

- developing a kinesthetic (sensory) awareness of your body positions during all movements.

- developing strong, yet relaxed, muscles and flexible joints.

- desiring to obtain good posture.

- having the discipline to continue what you have learned.

As you understand correct techniques, you can challenge yourself to try to use these positions in every total fitness component of your program (stretching, aerobics, step training, fitness walking and strength training exercises). At first you'll be thinking through the activity, but with persistent practice and desire you can exchange former faulty habits for safe, more complimentary ones. If you can attain a balanced standing posture, you've mastered this task already.

Dynamic Posture

Performing the aerobics or step training gesture and step patterns or the fitness walking will require you to take a different body position, or posture, than when you are standing stationary and poised. You are preparing dynamically to move in some direction through space (forward, backward, laterally, up, down). While preparing to move through space, the broader your base of support, the lower your center of gravity (weight center) becomes. This allows for better balance so you can move quickly and more efficiently in any direction.

Posture is where a total program for physical fitness begins.

FIGURE 4.4   Characteristics of Good Posture

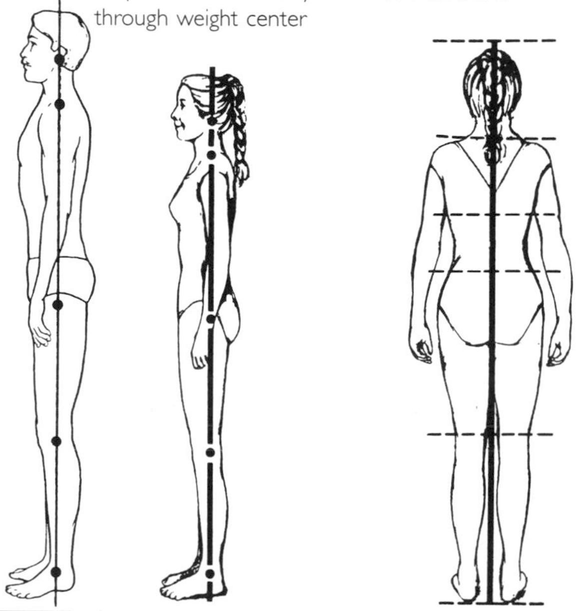

SIDE VIEW

Line of gravity passes:

1. Through tip of ear
2. Through center of shoulders
3. Slightly behind center of hip
4. Behind kneecap
5. In front of ankle joint
6. Perpendicular vertically through weight center

1. Head is up

2. Chin is parallel to floor

3. Ear is above middle of shoulder

4. Tip of shoulder is over hip joint

5. Shoulders are relaxed and down

6. Chest and rib cage are lifted

7. Abdomen is flat

8. Pelvis is balanced; front of pelvis and thigh are in a continuous line

9. Knees are unlocked or slightly flexed

10. Feet are parallel; body weight is centered between heel and toe and carried on outer half of feet

BACK VIEW

Line of gravity passes through:

1. Mid-head
2. Mid-trunk
3. Mid-waist
4. Mid-ankle

1. Head is erect
2. Body is symmetrical

3. Shoulders are level

4. Spine is straight

5. Hips are level

6. Legs are straight

7. Feet are parallel; toes are pointing forward

8. Weight is distributed equally on both feet and toward outer half of each foot

Practice

For your total daily well-being, good posture must become important enough to you to make it a life-long endeavor. Are you sitting correctly while reading how to improve your posture?

Daily practice is required for good posture to become an integral part of you. Good posture is established only through discipline. Setting aside time to do exercises such as those that follow to encourage good posture and develop strength and flexibility, accompanied by constant attention to posture throughout your daily living tasks, will turn this into reality. You can improve as you move — all day, every day.

EXERCISES TO PROMOTE POSTURAL AWARENESS

Exercising the antigravity muscles is a fundamental part of any total physical fitness conditioning program. To develop and then maintain a good posture, these muscles have to be:

- *strong* enough to perform their functions.
- *flexible* enough to allow a variety of movements.
- *relaxed* enough to perform with ease.

Therefore, establishing a program of *strength* exercises for the abdomen, lower back, hip, thigh, and calf areas will help you to obtain a balanced pelvic alignment and provide the means for efficient and painless movement. As mentioned, each joint involved has to be flexible enough to permit the full range of movement possible from these groups of antigravity muscles so that any new position can be maintained properly. The following exercises will help you develop joint *flexibility* of the antigravity muscle groups needed to maintain correct postures. Establishing a *program of relaxation* will assist with ease of performance while moving or while motionless.

The best exercise you can do for yourself is both a physical and mental one: *Become aware of correct postural technique with every move you make.* Then practice this physical and mental conditioning constantly until it becomes a habit, until it becomes you.

Elbows Wide 'n Close

To understand the awareness of "space between shoulder blades" *contracted* and then *widely*

stretched, keeping the chest raised for either direction (see Figure 4.5):

1. Clasp your hands loosely behind your head (a). Do not tightly lace fingers behind the neck. Pulling on the cervical spine is not a good body position. Keep your *elbows out and high*, shoulders down, and your chin parallel to the floor. (4 counts)

2. Exhale, and widen the space between your shoulder blades by bringing elbows *together* in front of your nose (b). (Hold for 4 counts)

3. Inhale, and return *elbows wide* to the sides (a). (4 counts)

4. Exhale and pull your elbows *up and back* (not shown), tightly contracting the space between your shoulder blades. (Hold 4 counts)

5. Inhale and return *elbows wide* (a) to the sides. (4 counts)

6. For variety, again attempt to touch elbows together, first *in front of forehead* and *below the chin*, maintaining the good posture position.

Cues: "Elbows out and high, together, wide, up and back, wide."

FIGURE 4.5   Elbows Wide 'n Close

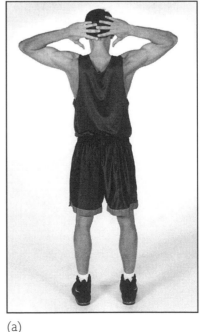 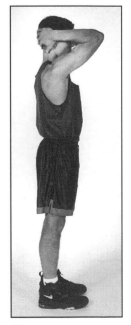

(a)   (b)

Rib Lifter

To establish awareness of the all-important position of "chest high" (and not sagging), this exercise (Figure 4.6) will help to isolate and stretch the intercostal (rib) muscles:

1. Stand in correct alignment, with your *arms forward* and *parallel* to the ground. Place your thumbs and index fingers of each hand together, hands forward, palms down (a). (4 counts)

2. Bend your elbows, bring your arms back, and place your palms parallel to the ground above your breast, with your *thumbs* snugly *under the armpits* and elbows held wide and parallel to the ground (b). (4 counts)

3. Without lifting your shoulders or bending forward, *lift your entire rib section as high as you can.* Breathe deeply, inhale, and exhale. (8 counts)

4. Now *lift* your elbow high and *stretch* rib cage on the one side (c). (4 counts)

5. *Lower* raised elbow to shoulder level. (4 counts)

6. Repeat with lifting and lowering of other elbow. (8 counts)

7. Repeat *raising both* together (d). Lower. (8 counts)

Cues: "Stand; thumbs under armpits; lift ribs, breathe and stretch; lower; repeat other side; repeat both; lower."

FIGURE 4.6 Rib Lifter

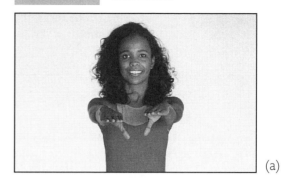

(a)

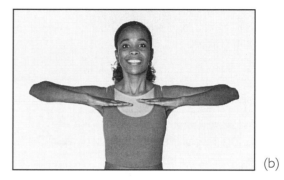

(b)

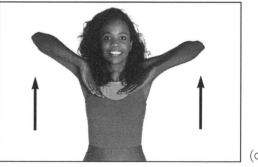

(c)

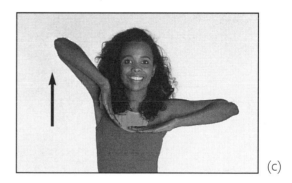

(d)

Reaching Correctly

To establish awareness in keeping the *shoulders back and down* as you perform arm movements that are forward and upward (Figure 4.7):

1. *Stand* in correct alignment. Place the back of your left hand on your central lower back and pelvic girdle area (a). (4 counts)

2. Slowly *raise* your right arm forward and in front of your body above your head, keeping your lower arm and hand stationary, your elbow still flexed (b). (4 counts)

3. Slowly *lower* your arm to its original position in standing alignment. (4 counts)

4. Place the back of your right hand on your central lower back, and slowly *raise and lower* your left arm as before (not shown). (8 counts)

5. With both arms lowered and both hands resting lightly on your thighs, slowly *raise both arms* in front of your body and above your head in the same manner in which each was raised (c). (4 counts)

6. Slowly *lower* to original position. (4 counts)

7. Repeat all, once again. (24 counts)

Cues: "Stand; raise one and lower; raise opposite and lower; raise both and lower."

FIGURE 4.7 **Reaching Correctly**

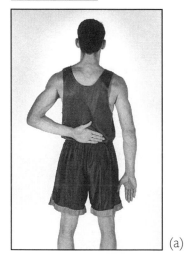

(a)

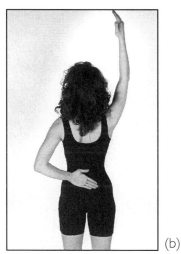

(b)

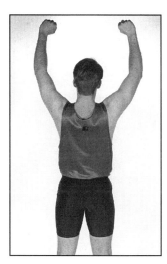

(c)

Correct Lifting and Lowering

To protect your muscles and joints (especially the lower back) from undue strain or fatigue, proper technique in these areas *must* become second nature to you. Disciplined practice of correct techniques *now* will establish good habits for the rest of your life. The leg muscles are very strong, whereas the back muscles are relatively weak. All heavy lifting should be done by stabilizing the back in an erect position and making the legs provide the necessary power (Figure 4.8).

1. Get as close as possible to the object, using a forward-stride position. The object should be in front of you if you are using two hands (e.g., step-bench) or beside you if you are using one hand (e.g., luggage). Keeping your back straight and your pelvis tucked, bend at the hips, knees, and ankles to lower your body. Lower directly downward, only as much as necessary (keeping your head high and buttocks low).

2. Place both arms well under or around the weight center of the load. Lift vertically upward in a slow, steady movement by *extending your leg muscles*. Keep the object close to your weight center (Figure 4.8). Reverse the procedure to lower the object.

Do not bend over from your hips (head low, buttocks high) and force your back muscles to lift the load (Figure 4.9).

FIGURE 4.9

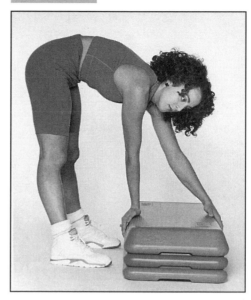

Incorrect lifting position.

Correct Carrying

1. Keep the object close to your weight center.
2. Separate the load when feasible, and carry half in each hand/arm (Figure 4.10).

FIGURE 4.8

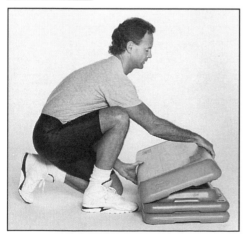

Correct lifting position.

FIGURE 4.10

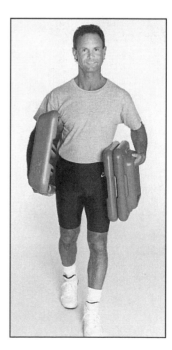

Correct carrying position.

Goal Setting Challenge

Set a goal to start looking good throughout your *entire* day by becoming aware of, and improving, your position in every type of physical activity you do.

Developing Goal Scripts for Chapter 4

DIRECTIONS: Write complete sentences for each segment below. Combine your responses to all four segments. This goal script is designed around your needs and choices. Read it (or make an audiotape and play it) twice daily, morning and evening, until you master it.

1 State one goal in positive, *present-tense* language. Ask yourself, "What will I experience — see, hear, taste, smell, feel — in regard to the results? Keep in mind that all powerful goals use the SMART formula: specific, measurable, achievable, realistic, timely.

_____

_____

2 State your *pleasure-value reasons*. Ask yourself, "Why am I totally committed to achieving this goal? What am I choosing to feel?"

_____

_____

3 State your *pain-avoidance value reasons*. Ask yourself, "What painful values do I choose to avoid feeling?"

_____

_____

4 State *immediate action(s)* you can take in the next 24 hours. Use positive, present-tense verbs such as *choose* and verbs ending with "ing."

_____

_____

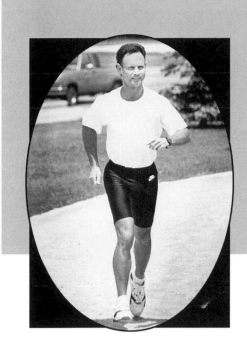

Fitness Testing

5

The next step in the journey toward achieving and then maintaining physical fitness for a lifetime involves establishing your current fitness starting point, using scientific test and assessment procedures. Clearly knowing yourself in terms of your past history, risk factors, and present physical status will assist you in developing a lifetime fitness plan. It will enable you to set realistically and safely achievable short-term fitness goals and also will provide the basis for motivating you continually to adhere to the program you do establish to achieve your long-range and lifetime fitness goals.

You initially may find it painful to realize that you are out of shape and test poorly on a laboratory or field stress test. No one wants to see or hear scientific results that are inferior or below the norm. Having the courage and determination to find out just where you are at the outset and then, with time and dedication, progressing to the point at which your post-assessment test numbers represent an excellent state of fitness and well-being is motivating, however.

In most instances specific fitness testing is appropriate only after obtaining a medical history. Screening may uncover any potential problems and determine if you should be considered for a specific exercise prescription. Most course settings require prescreening, or a thorough medical exam if you have any limitations or known risk factors.

UNDERSTANDING FITNESS ASSESSMENTS

The purpose of an initial pre-course fitness assessment is to establish a baseline of information to which later changes can be compared. Assessment principles include the following:

1. Nearly all assessment protocols result in *estimated* values for the fitness component being measured. Therefore the testing is mainly an effective way to measure improvement in your performance over time, not an absolutely correct physiologic measurement or comparison.

2. By following consistent procedures of testing (using the same test, same person administering it, same instrument, same time of day), you are more likely to have accurate measurements over time.

3. Results are recorded for comparison purposes. The person being tested should understand these values and ask questions as needed to ensure understanding.

MEASURING AEROBIC CAPACITY

Preassessment of your current status by a thorough physical fitness exam will include measurement of your heart's response to increasing amounts of exercise by measuring your ability to use oxygen. Physical fitness can and should be measured in one of two ways at least every 3 years:

● A laboratory physical fitness test.
● A field test administered by you and a friend.

Laboratory Physical Fitness Test

A properly conducted treadmill stress test is done to check the precise condition of your heart.[1] Physical fitness and health are different, and the treadmill stress ECG helps to make that distinction.[2]

Prior to a treadmill stress test, you will be screened thoroughly. The screening will consist of: (a) a brief history-taking and physical exam during which the technician will listen to your heart and lungs; (b) a check for the use of drugs (e.g., various heart and hypertensive medications) known to affect the ECG; (c) a check for history of any congenital or acquired heart disorders; and (d) an evaluation of the resting ECG.

This screening and background check will help to determine your risk factors. A risk factor is a feature in a person's heredity, background, or present lifestyle that increases the likelihood of developing coronary heart disease. If no risk factors are present, an exercise test usually is not necessary below age 35 if the guidelines mentioned in Chapter 1 are followed. If symptoms of heart, lung, or metabolic disease are present, a maximum stress test is recommended for individuals of any age prior to the onset of a vigorous exercise program, followed by a test every 2 years.[3]

SUBMAXIMAL TESTING

Submaximal testing is accomplished by means of a physical fitness test (stress test) on a treadmill. Electrocardiogram leads transmit and record electrical (heart) impulses that are read on a machine and recorded on a strip of paper. You are tested to only approximately 150 beats per minute, not to exhaustion.

The ECG electrodes with leads are circular rubber discs with wires attached to them. The discs are glued onto the chest and back at key locations so various "pictures" of your heart, from different angles and sides, all can be recorded at once. Usually between seven and ten electrodes are applied, depending on the laboratory's procedures or the individual's specific needs.

You probably will be asked to walk at a pace of 3.3 miles per hour (90 meters per minute) on the treadmill. The grade will begin flat and will increase slowly in gradation, as if you were walking up a hill. Every minute the "hill" will become steeper and more difficult to climb. When your heart rate reaches 150 beats per minute, a record is made of the amount of time it took you to arrive at that reading. Then, through an indirect method of extrapolation (projection of maximum results through having tested many others the same way in the past), your fitness ability is estimated.

Basically, the longer your heart rate takes to reach 150 beats per minute, the more fit you are; the shorter it takes, the less fit you are. Sub-maximal fitness testing usually is used with individuals who know of no outstanding limitations and who are interested in starting a total fitness program.

MAXIMAL TESTING

Maximal testing procedures are administered if an individual's need is more specific, as for diagnostic or research purposes. Maximum testing reveals directly how much oxygen you use, because you are tested to exhaustion. The exhaustion point is when you start to get markedly fatigued. Some researchers believe that maximum laboratory testing is the only conclusive form to use.

If you are over age 35, you should start an aerobic exercise program by first seeing your doctor and then taking a monitored laboratory fitness test. Individuals with known cardiovascular, pulmonary, or metabolic disease should have a maximum stress test prior to beginning vigorous exercise at any age. These people and those whose exercise tests are abnormal should get a stress test annually.

Field Tests of Fitness

You may not have immediate access to a laboratory and qualified physiologists to monitor the results recorded through the treadmill method. Therefore, field tests have been developed to help you assess your own physical fitness by determining your current aerobic capacity. This testing is conducted easily in a fitness class setting.

The following information and Figures 5.1, 5.2, and 5.3 were developed from Dr. Kenneth Cooper's book, *The Aerobics Program for Total Well-Being.*[4] You can administer Cooper's 12-Minute Test, 1.5-Mile Test, and 3-Mile Walking Test by yourself or with the help of a friend. You should assess your cardiorespiratory endurance using one of these tests before you begin your aerobic exercise program and reassess your cardiorespiratory efficiency 8 weeks later. As aerobic exercise becomes a lifetime activity for you, an ongoing assessment should be done every 2 months, and your results compared with those from your first assessment. This also will help you set continual, lifelong, specific physical fitness goals.

As guidelines for field-testing:

1. If you have been physically inactive previously, participate in 1 to 2 weeks of walking or slow jogging before undertaking any of Cooper's tests.

2. Wear loose clothing in which you can sweat freely, and a sport shoe that conforms to the guidelines suggested in Chapter 3.

3. Determine first which field test you plan to take. You can choose running with time or distance as the stopping point; or fitness walking with your distance covered as the stopping point.
   - If time is the stopping point, take the 12-Minute Test.
   - If distance is the stopping point, take the 1.5-Mile Test, or 3-Mile Walking Test.
   - If you believe rather strongly that you are really out of shape, take the 12-Minute Test because you run for this amount of time only. (You might take 20 minutes to complete 1.5 miles or 60 minutes to complete 3 miles.)

4. Have a stopwatch or a second-hand on your watch, or be close to a timer.

5. Immediately before performing the test, spend 5 to 10 minutes warming up your muscles (see Chapter 6).

6. Have a partner record your data (as the time it takes or laps or distance).

7. Run or walk (or a combination) as quickly as you can for the 12-Minute Test or 1.5-Mile Test. Perform the Walking Test by covering 3 miles in the fastest time possible *without running*. These are all-out tests of endurance.

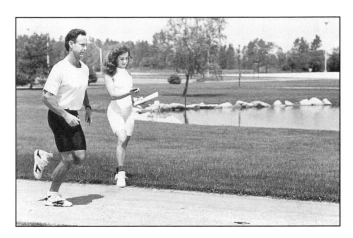

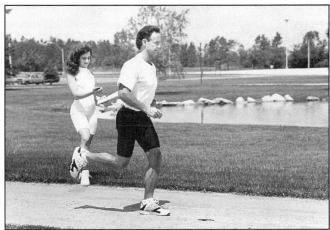

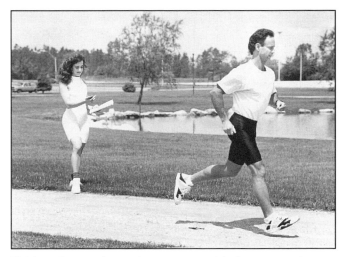

Field-testing to determine your aerobic fitness starting point.

FIGURE 5.1   Cooper's 12-Minute Walking/Running Test

Fitness Category		Age (Years)					
		13-19	20-29	30-39	40-49	50-59	60 +
		Distance (Miles) Covered in 12 Minutes					
I. Very Poor	(men)	<1.30	<1.22	<1.18	<1.14	<1.03	< .87
	(women)	<1.0	< .96	< .94	< .88	< .84	< .78
II. Poor	(men)	1.30-1.37	1.22-1.31	1.18-1.30	1.14-1.24	1.03-1.16	.87-1.02
	(women)	1.00-1.18	.96-1.11	.95-1.05	.88- .98	.84- .93	.78- .86
III. Fair	(men)	1.38-1.56	1.32-1.49	1.31-1.45	1.25-1.39	1.17-1.30	1.03-1.20
	(women)	1.19-1.29	1.12-1.22	1.06-1.18	.99-1.11	.94-1.05	.87- .98
IV. Good	(men)	1.57-1.72	1.50-1.64	1.46-1.56	1.40-1.53	1.31-1.44	1.21-1.32
	(women)	1.30-1.43	1.23-1.34	1.19-1.29	1.12-1.24	1.06-1.18	.99-1.09
V. Excellent	(men)	1.73-1.86	1.65-1.76	1.57-1.69	1.54-1.65	1.45-1.58	1.33-1.55
	(women)	1.44-1.51	1.35-1.45	1.30-1.39	1.25-1.34	1.19-1.30	1.10-1.18
VI. Superior	(men)	>1.87	>1.77	>1.70	>1.66	>1.59	>1.56
	(women)	>1.52	>1.46	>1.40	>1.35	>1.31	>1.19

< = less than;   > = more than.

PRE-TEST

Start Time: _____   Stop Time: _____   Distance Covered: _____

Circle Fitness Category: Very Poor   Poor   Fair   Good   Excellent   Superior

COURSE GOAL: _____

POST-TEST

Start Time: _____   Stop Time: _____   Distance Covered: _____

Circle Fitness Category: Very Poor   Poor   Fair   Good   Excellent   Superior

2-MONTH GOAL: _____

FIGURE 5.2   Cooper's 1.5-Mile Run/Walk Test

Fitness Category		Age (Years) 13-19	20-29	30-39	40-49	50-59	60 +
		Time (Minutes)					
I. Very Poor	(men)	>15:31	>16:01	>16:31	>17:31	>19:01	>20:01
	(women)	>18:31	>19:01	>19:31	>20:01	>20:31	>21:01
II. Poor	(men)	12:11-15:30	14:01-16:00	14:44-16:30	15:36-17:30	17:01-19:00	19:01-20:00
	(women)	16:55-18:30	18:31-19:00	19:01-19:30	19:31-20:00	20:01-20:30	21:00-21:31
III. Fair	(men)	10:49-12:10	12:01-14:00	12:31-14:45	13:01-15:35	14:31-17:00	16:16-19:00
	(women)	14:31-16:54	15:55-18:30	16:31-19:00	17:31-19:30	19:01-20:00	19:31-20:30
IV. Good	(men)	9:41-10:48	10:46-12:00	11:01-12:30	11:31-13:00	12:31-14:30	14:00-16:15
	(women)	12:30-14:30	13:31-15:54	14:31-16:30	15:56-17:30	16:31-19:00	17:31-19:30
V. Excellent	(men)	8:37- 9:40	9:45-10:45	10:00-11:00	10:30-11:30	11:00-12:30	11:15-13:59
	(women)	11:50-12:29	12:30-13:30	13:00-14:30	13:45-15:55	14:30-16:30	16:30-17:30
VI. Superior	(men)	< 8:37	< 9:45	<10:00	<10:30	<11:00	<11:15
	(women)	<11:50	<12:30	<13:00	<13:45	<14:30	<16:30

< = less than;   > = more than.

From *The Aerobics Program For Total Well-Being*, by Kenneth H. Cooper. © Copyright 1982 by Kenneth H. Cooper. Reprinted by permission of the publisher, Bantam-Doubleday-Dell, New York, NY 10103.

PRE-TEST

Check off laps (e.g., 14 for 190-yard track; 21 for 126-yard track):

1 - 2 - 3 - 4 - 5 - 6 - 7 - 8 - 9 - 10 - 11 - 12 - 13 - 14 - 15 - 16 - 17 - 18 - 19 - 20 - 21

Time: _____ OR:

Record here if using an open roadway.

     Stop Time: _____

   − Start Time: _____

     Time: _____

Circle Fitness Category:

Very Poor   Poor   Fair

Good   Excellent   Superior

COURSE GOAL: _____

POST-TEST

Check off laps (e.g., 14 for 190-yard track; 21 for 126-yard track):

1 - 2 - 3 - 4 - 5 - 6 - 7 - 8 - 9 - 10 - 11 - 12 - 13 - 14 - 15 - 16 - 17 - 18 - 19 - 20 - 21

Time: _____ OR:

Record here if using an open roadway.

     Stop Time: _____

   − Start Time: _____

     Time: _____

Circle Fitness Category:

Very Poor   Poor   Fair

Good   Excellent   Superior

2-MONTH GOAL: _____

| FIGURE 5.3 | Cooper's 3-Mile Walking Test (No Running) |

Fitness Category		Age (Years)					
		13-19	20-29	30-39	40-49	50-59	60 +
		Time (Minutes)					
I. Very Poor	(men)	>45:00	>46:00	>49:00	>52:00	>55:00	>60:00
	(women)	>47:00	>48:00	>51:00	>54:00	>57:00	>63:00
II. Poor	(men)	41:01-45:00	42:01-46:00	44:31-49:00	47:01-52:00	50:01-55:00	54:01-60:00
	(women)	43:01-47:00	44:01-48:00	46:31-51:00	49:01-54:00	52:01-57:00	57:01-63:00
III. Fair	(men)	37:31-41:00	38:31-42:00	40:01-44:30	42:01-47:00	45:01-50:00	48:01-54:00
	(women)	39:31-43:00	40:31-44:00	42:01-46:30	44:01-49:00	47:01-52:00	51:01-57:00
IV. Good	(men)	33:00-37:30	34:00-38:30	35:00-40:00	36:30-42:00	39:00-45:00	41:00-48:00
	(women)	35:00-39:30	36:00-40:30	37:30-42:00	39:00-44:00	42:00-47:00	45:00-51:00
V. Excellent	(men)	<33:00	<34:00	<35:00	<36:30	<39:00	<41:00
	(women)	<35:00	<36:00	<37:30	<39:00	<42:00	<45:00

< = less than;   > = more than.

From *The Aerobics Program For Total Well-Being*, by Kenneth H. Cooper. © Copyright 1982 by Kenneth H. Cooper. Reprinted by permission of the publisher, Bantam-Doubleday-Dell, New York, NY 10103.

PRE-TEST

Check off laps (e.g., 28 for 190-yard track; 42 for 126-yard track):

1 - 2 - 3 - 4 - 5 - 6 - 7 - 8 - 9 - 10 - 11 - 12 - 13 - 14 - 15 - 16 - 17 - 18 - 19 - 20 - 21 - 22 - 23 - 24 - 25
26 - 27 - 28 - 29 - 30 - 31 - 32 - 33 - 34 - 35 - 36 - 37 - 38 - 39 - 40 - 41 - 42

Time: _____ OR:

Record here if using an open roadway.

    Stop Time: _____

   – Start Time: _____

      Time: _____

Circle Fitness Category:

Very Poor   Poor   Fair

Good   Excellent

COURSE GOAL: _____

POST-TEST

Check off laps (e.g., 28 for 190-yard track; 42 for 126-yard track):

1 - 2 - 3 - 4 - 5 - 6 - 7 - 8 - 9 - 10 - 11 - 12 - 13 - 14 - 15 - 16 - 17 - 18 - 19 - 20 - 21 - 22 - 23 - 24 - 25
26 - 27 - 28 - 29 - 30 - 31 - 32 - 33 - 34 - 35 - 36 - 37 - 38 - 39 - 40 - 41 - 42

Time: _____ OR:

Record here if using an open roadway.

    Stop Time: _____

   – Start Time: _____

      Time: _____

Circle Fitness Category:

Very Poor   Poor   Fair

Good   Excellent

8. When you stop, identify precisely the distance covered in miles and tenths of miles or time you took, and have your partner record it.

9. Cool down by first walking slowly for several minutes, and then finish by doing cool-down stretching.

10. Interpret your results for the specific test you used, in the forms provided in Figures 5.1, 5.2, or 5.3. At the conclusion of your course, re-assess your fitness. What changes did you experience from the pre-test to the post-test?

For some beginners the "good" performance level is high. Do not be discouraged. You will be pleased with your improvement as you participate in a regular aerobics program.

FITNESS FOR LIFE

Attaining a level of physical fitness labeled "good" or "high" (lab tests), or "good," "excellent," or "superior" (field tests) does not mean you have achieved a finished product or goal. Instead, you have found a method of getting in shape that must be continued for the rest of your life. If you discontinue your program completely, all your aerobic gains will be lost in 10 weeks.[5]

The quest for personal fitness must result in a complete change in lifestyle. You must prioritize and program exercise into your busy weekly schedule for the rest of your life. A "yo-yo" concept of a 10-week class now and maybe one a year later just doesn't maintain fitness and a healthy heart.

You have just completed assessing your aerobic capacity. With this information, you can establish your cardiovascular fitness goal for the course, or for time intervals after the course is over.

The quest for personal fitness must result in a complete change in lifestyle.

Goal Setting Challenge

 Write one fitness goal to be achieved by the end of this course. Truly stretch yourself and your potential in regard to what you are actually capable of achieving.

Developing Goal Scripts for Chapter 5

DIRECTIONS: Write complete sentences for each segment below. Combine your responses to all four segments. This goal script is designed around your needs and choices. Read it (or make an audiotape and play it) twice daily, morning and evening, until you master it.

1 State one goal in positive, *present-tense* language. Ask yourself, "What will I experience — see, hear, taste, smell, feel — in regard to the results? Keep in mind that all powerful goals use the SMART formula: specific, measurable, achievable, realistic, timely.

_____

_____

2 State your *pleasure-value reasons*. Ask yourself, "Why am I totally committed to achieving this goal? What am I choosing to feel?"

_____

_____

3 State your *pain-avoidance value reasons*. Ask yourself, "What painful values do I choose to avoid feeling?"

_____

_____

4 State *immediate action(s)* you can take in the next 24 hours. Use positive, present-tense verbs such as *choose* and verbs ending with "ing."

_____

_____

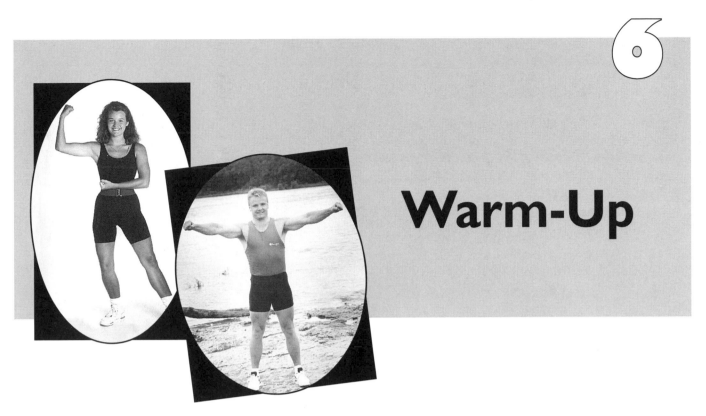

Warm-Up

The foundation for understanding physical fitness has been set. The terminology and criteria have been defined. The sensory-based components of motivation have been explored. You've become aware of the key questions to ask so you can set powerful, life-changing goals for every phase of your program. Strong encouragement has been (and will continue to be) given constantly to facilitate setting SMART goals — short-, medium-, or long-term — whatever works best for you. You've been informed about the risk and safety factors involved and good positioning that must be incorporated into all parts of your program to see results that last! And you've been given several fitness testing procedures for estimating your cardiovascular starting point.

Now we can build upon this base with principles and techniques that represent a safe, beneficial, and fun total fitness workout session.[1, 2, 3, 4, 5, 6, 7, 8, 9, 10] The first of these program segments is the warm-up.

LIMBERING EXERCISES

The warm-up begins with activities that are active, medium-to-low-level, rhythmic, limbering, standing, range-of-motion types of exercises that raise the body's core temperature slightly, initiate muscular

movements, and prepare you for more strenuous moves to come. Examples such as step-touch with low arm-curl swings, strides with sweeping punches (shown in the chapter opening photos), and other smooth, sweeping motions of low intensity (Figure 6.1) are good to initiate the warm-up. The time-frame is approximately 3 to 5 minutes.

FIGURE 6.1   Step-Out Wide and Squat

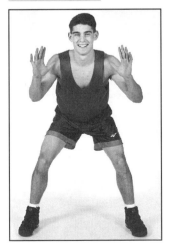 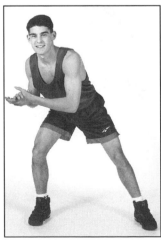

(a) Step-out wide and squat. Hold.

(b) Side-clap left, side clap right. (4 counts)

Note: **All techniques are photographed and described by the "mirroring technique," in which the words and movement are to be done exactly as shown.**

STATIC STRETCHING

Following the initial warm-up exercises, slow-sustained, static stretching is performed, because the muscles, tendons, ligaments, and joints are now loose and pliable. Static stretching is done from head to toe (Figures 6.2-6.14).

Static stretching is probably the most popular, easiest, and safest form of stretching. It involves stretching a muscle or muscle group gradually to the point of limitation, then holding that position for approximately 15 seconds. The stretch is repeated to the opposite side. Several repetitions of each stretch are performed. Static stretching is recommended when muscles are warm — after the initial active phase of the warm-up, and later after intense physical activity.

Breathing should be continuous. Your entire system, especially your working muscles, constantly needs oxygen. Holding your breath and turning red is never acceptable technique. While performing the warm-up or cool-down stretching (or any strengthening exercise), you should *exhale when you stretch*, by puckering your lips and breathing out, and *inhale when you relax your muscles*. Cue yourself: "Breathe out and stretch; breathe in and relax." The timeframe suggested for the warm-up stretching segment is approximately 5 minutes.

STATIC STRETCHING MOVES

FIGURE 6.2   Lateral Neck Stretch

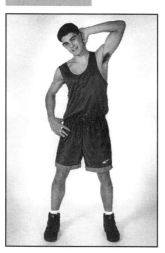

Drop head to L side and press with R palm, keeping elbow high. Stabilize with L hand on hip. Hold. (8 counts) Reverse R side. (8 counts)

FIGURE 6.3   Trunk Sideward Lean

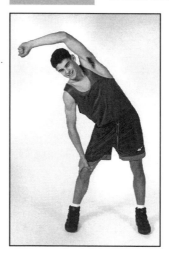

Sliding L hand down to L thigh, lean L; R hand and arm reach and stretch, close over head. Hold. (8 counts) Reverse R side. (8 counts)

FIGURE 6.4   Shoulder Circles

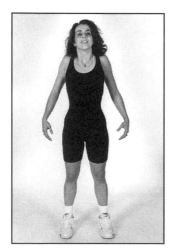

Up, back, down, forward; or alternate, one at a time. (4 counts in each direction)

FIGURE 6.5   Arm Sweeps

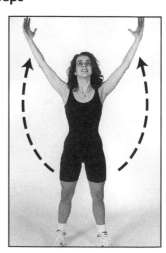

Arms low and center; wide and palms up; raise, reach high. (8 counts) Reverse. (8 counts)

STATIC STRETCHING MOVES

FIGURE 6.6   **Shoulder / Upper Back Stretch**

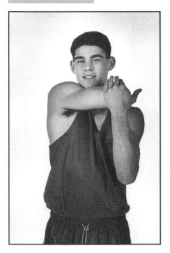

(a) Bring L upper arm under chin, keeping L elbow shoulder high; press L elbow toward you with R palm. Hold. (8 counts)

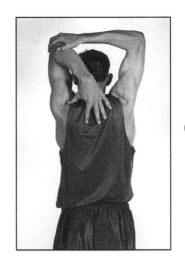

(b) Raise L arm/elbow above head, placing L palm on center back; raise R arm, framing head, R elbow kept high; R palm presses L elbow backward. Hold. (8 counts) Reverse (a), then (b). (16 counts)

FIGURE 6.7   **Chest Stretch**

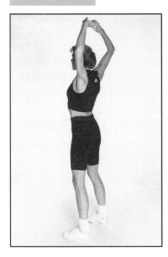

(a) Grasp hands very high, elbows bent, press back, and hold. (8 counts)

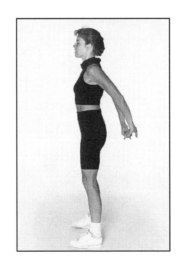

(b) Grasp hands low, behind back, lift and hold. (8 counts)

FIGURE 6.8   **Low Back Stretch**

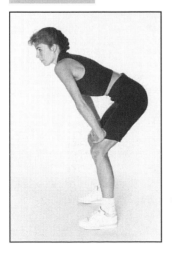

(a) Feet apart, hands on thighs, flatten back. Hold. (8 counts)

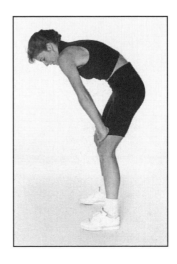

(b) Now round lower back upward, contract abdominals, tuck buttocks under hips. Hold. (8 counts)

STATIC STRETCHING MOVES

FIGURE 6.9 Inner Thigh Stretch

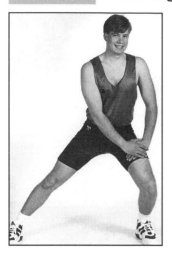

Feet apart/toes forward, shift weight/hips R; flex R knee over R toe. Hold. (8/16 counts) Reverse.

FIGURE 6.10 Hip Flexor Stretch

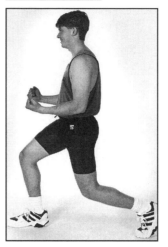

Forward/back stride, feet forward, fists at waist; firmly tuck buttocks under hips, flex and lower front knee. Contract hip flexors by now bringing back knee forward, with weight on ball of back foot and forward foot. Hold. (8/16 counts) Reverse. (8/16 counts)

FIGURE 6.11 Hamstring Stretch

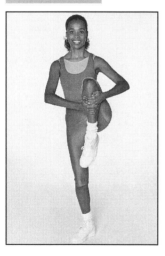

Weight L and turned out; encircle R knee and bring to chest, keeping spine upright. Hold. (8 counts) Reverse. (8 counts)

FIGURE 6.12 Calf Stretch

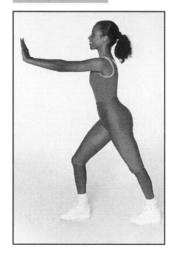

Immediately step backward with same leg held, feet in forward/backward stride; *bend* front knee just over toes, keeping back foot flat on floor. Straight arm forward press. Hold. (8 counts) Walk through and reverse. (8 counts)

FIGURE 6.13 Quadriceps and Iliopsoas Stretch

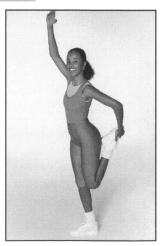

L foot turned outward carrying weight, bend R knee/leg backward, grasping shoestring area with R hand; L hand high and back for balance. Keeping knee pointing down and legs together, bring heel close to buttocks. Hold. (8 counts) Reverse. (8 counts)

STATIC STRETCHING MOVES

FIGURE 6.14 **Ankle Stretch**

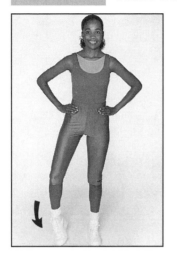 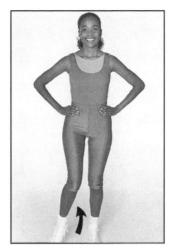

Static stretching is probably the most popular, easiest, and safest form of stretching.

(a) Weight on R foot and ball of L. Circle L ankle, stretching out, back, in, forward. (8 counts)

(b) Reverse. (8 counts)

Repeat, weight L stretching R ankle. (16 counts)

MONITORING PROGRESS

At the conclusion of the warm-up and stretching from head to toe, determine how hard you are working (intensity) by taking your pulse. The pulse tends to be in the range of 90–120 beats per minute (bpm), and the accompanying number of how you feel on the Borg Scale Ratings of Perceived Exertion should be approximately a "2" (see Chapter 1, Figure 1.5).

Goal Setting Challenge

 Immediately after each exercise session, take time to record your progress and gains in a journal. A sample page is located in Chapter 15.

 Record any setbacks also. It will give you a visual blueprint on how successfully you are accomplishing a variety of short-term goals, and how you can do so again in the future. Include today's date, exercise varieties, time duration, short-term goal set, new achievement today, and your thoughts and feelings. Enjoy the process of changing.

Developing Goal Scripts for Chapter 6

DIRECTIONS: Write complete sentences for each segment below. Combine your responses to all four segments. This goal script is designed around your needs and choices. Read it (or make an audiotape and play it) twice daily, morning and evening, until you master it.

1 State one goal in positive, *present-tense* language. Ask yourself, "What will I experience — see, hear, taste, smell, feel — in regard to the results? Keep in mind that all powerful goals use the SMART formula: specific, measurable, achievable, realistic, timely.

_____

_____

2 State your *pleasure-value reasons.* Ask yourself, "Why am I totally committed to achieving this goal? What am I choosing to feel?"

_____

_____

3 State your *pain-avoidance value reasons.* Ask yourself, "What painful values do I choose to avoid feeling?"

_____

_____

4 State *immediate action(s)* you can take in the next 24 hours. Use positive, present-tense verbs such as *choose* and verbs ending with "ing."

_____

_____

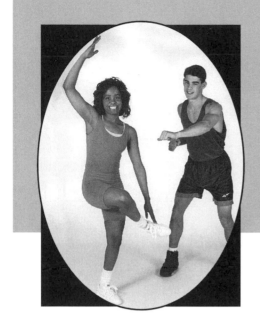

Aerobic Exercise:
Aerobics (Option 1)

The aerobic segment of your fitness program can include any activity that promotes the supply and use of oxygen, provided that the aerobic exercise criteria established in Chapter 1 are followed. The aerobic exercise modalities presented in this book are *aerobics* (presented in this chapter), *step training* (Chapter 8), and *fitness walking* and *jumping rope* (Chapter 9).

PRINCIPLES OF AEROBICS

In addition to how often (frequency), how much work (heartbeats per minute/intensity), and how long to work out (duration of time per session), the concept of *impact* has to be considered when determining your fitness program.

Basic step movements in aerobics have changed considerably since the origin of the activity. These changes have centered on reducing and preventing injury, with the primary focus on the amount of vertical force exerted on the feet as they contact the floor surface and how this stress subsequently effects the musculoskeletal system.

Early programs included many steps and gestures with great bodily elevation and corresponding great compression upon foot contact with the floor. Research has given the aerobics enthusiast a variety of safe alternatives regarding impact and movement possibilities.

High-Impact Aerobics (HIA)

High-impact aerobics (HIA) involves steps and gestures in which both feet may be off the floor at the same time briefly. This step movement selection results in great force exerted when the foot meets the floor surface. This force is absorbed by the landing, floor surface, shoes, orthotics (if worn), and musculoskeletal system (muscles, tendons, ligaments, joints, and bones).

Several examples of basic movements that are considered high-impact are jogging, hopping, and jumping. A few characteristics of high-impact aerobics are:

- Music between 130 and 160 beats per minute (bpm).
- Faster music, smaller moves.
- Slower music, greater range of motion.
- Landing through toe/ball/heel.
- Avoiding more than eight repetitions (reps) on one limb.
- Strengthening anterior tibialis (shin area).
- Strengthening hamstrings.
- Limited to every other day.
- Higher intensity = $>VO_2$ max.
- Moderate intensity > fat utilization.[1]

Note: High-impact aerobics is generally *not recommended* for:

- Individuals who obviously are in poor condition or out of shape, especially obese people.
- Anyone who is susceptible to specific injuries (such as shin splints) caused by, or likely to be aggravated by, upward impacts on the feet.
- Women in the latter stages of pregnancy, who usually have loosened joints.
- Individuals who are incontinent (unable to control urination).
- Individuals who are uncomfortable with high-impact steps.[2]

Low-Impact Aerobics (LIA)

Low-impact aerobics (LIA) involves steps and gestures that produce less force when the feet strike the floor than those in high-impact movements. In LIA great control over the landing and force of foot impact is present, because one foot is in contact with the floor at all times.

Low-impact does not mean low-intensity! Cardiorespiratory conditioning still can be achieved as long as you are working within the target heart rate training zone you've established. To help elevate your heart rate if it is not in your zone, place more emphasis on weight-bearing moves that lower your center of gravity. Deepening knee flexion (bending motions) that use the large leg and buttocks muscles (quadriceps and hamstrings, and gluteals) and gesture actions of the upper body are ways to accomplish this. Examples of low-impact moves are step-touch, lunge, grapevine, marching, and vigorous walking in place. Characteristics of low-impact aerobics are:

- Heart rate is kept in the target heart rate (THR) training zone.
- Moves can be modified if the THR is not maintained.
- Any music tempo can be utilized.
- With faster tempos, less space is covered.
- With slower tempos, more space is covered.
- Feet are kept closer to the ground to decrease impact.

In LIA great control over the landing and force of foot impact is present, because one foot is in contact with the floor at all times.

- Moves require traveling from side-to-side and forward-and-back so large muscles of legs and trunk are engaged continuously.
- Controlled, vigorous arm movements compensate for reduction in activity of the leg and back muscles when the height of hops and jumps is reduced. "Research has shown that up to 25% more work can be performed with the arms and legs combined, compared to work performed by the legs alone.[3]
- Arms are not used above shoulder level for extended periods. "Doing so necessitates extended isometric contractions of the arm and shoulder muscles and probably causes greater after-exercise soreness. In addition, holding the arms over the head raises blood pressure, and anyone with high blood pressure or a history of angina pectoralis should be discouraged from doing these movements.[4]
- Toes/knees are turned out, with wide legs.
  - Center of gravity is raised and lowered.
  - In lateral moves, legs are turned out.
  - Angle of knee flexion is 90°.
  - Vastus medialis (front, inner thigh) and hamstrings are strengthened.
- Adductor muscles are used for correct mechanics.[5]

Note: Low-impact aerobics (LIA) is generally *not recommended* for:

- Anyone who complains of knee discomfort during prolonged knee flexion.
- Individuals who have severely flattened or pronated feet. (Knee flexion, and some side-to-side movements in which one foot crosses in front of the other, tend to produce a shifting of the kneecap toward the outer side of the knee joint, which increases stress.)
- Well-conditioned, injury-free individuals who are unable to achieve their target heart rate, even in the most intense LIA program. (Although many instructors use LIA exclusively in the interest of safety, conventional high-impact choreography may be acceptable for these participants as long as they remain injury-free.[6])

Combination High-/Low-Impact Aerobics (CIA or Combo-Impact)

The combination style of choreography utilizes characteristics of both high- and low-impact movement and can be a safe and exciting blend. Combination high/low-impact choreography can be defined in two ways.[7]

1. *Routines that offer both a high-impact and a low-impact version of a movement.* Programs that offer both of these work best in classes with mixed fitness levels so individual participants can select the amount of impact appropriate for them. A beginner in the program, therefore, may choose to do the low-impact version, whereas an experienced dance-exerciser may feel more challenged by the high-impact movements.

2. *Routines combining a series of varied high-impact and a series of varied low-impact movements.* This style lends itself well to classes of experienced aerobics exercisers whose primary concern is to improve cardiorespiratory fitness while minimizing the risk of injury.

Combo-impact aerobics offers a wide range of choices and possibilities. It allows you to individualize how much physical stress you choose to experience safely at various times and stages of your life according to your fitness level, personal goals, and special interests. Especially if you are a beginner,

coming off an illness or injury, obese, older, or pregnant, you will want to choose the less biomechanically stressful low-impact movements. Athletes in training and well-conditioned, injury-free individuals may choose the high-impact movements and series more frequently, or even exclusively. As another option, they may wish to blend their HIA and LIA techniques into the *moderate-impact aerobic* (MIA) style explained in the next section.

The unique feature of a combination approach is that participants can choose from the various possibilities the impact that best fits their current lifestyle needs. Some people, of course, can never participate in the high-impact movements because of permanent physical limitations.

As illustrated by Figures 7.1-7.4, a three-step process for interpreting any high-impact steps into acceptable low-impact movement can be accomplished by:

1. Lowering the foot impact.
2. Increasing the arm movement.
3. Increasing the use of space.

Step 1 of this process minimizes the impact, and steps 2 and 3 increase the intensity of the movement. The idea is to change one element at a time. Combining a series of varied high-impact and a series of varied low-impact movements will produce fewer of the large upward impacts typical of a HIA program

FIGURE 7.1

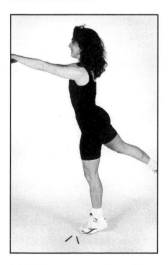

High-impact version of a lunge (momentarily airborne).

FIGURE 7.2

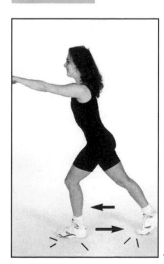

Lower impact by stepping backward or forward instead of jumping.

FIGURE 7.3

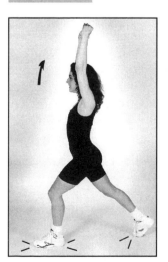

Increased intensity by raising arms above shoulders.

FIGURE 7.4

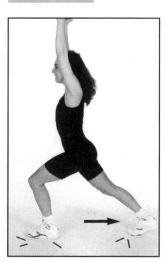

Increased use of space by reaching out farther.

and fewer of the large side-to-side impacts typical of many LIA programs. Keen attention to the beat of the music becomes important when converting high-impact movement to low impact movement, to ensure an injury-free workout. The sum total of all the stresses on the various vulnerable parts of the body is what determines whether injury occurs.

Moderate-Impact Aerobics (MIA)

The fourth and the newest alternative style of impact aerobics is called moderate-impact aerobics (MIA). It was designed as the result of laboratory and dance-exercise class research done at San Diego State University.[8] By adapting the gesture style (non-weight-bearing body parts) and foot impact, this choreographic style combines the best elements of both HIA and LIA, for movements that keep the intensity needed to maintain target heart rate while reducing foot-impact forces.

This key technique is called *plyometric*.[9] At least one foot remains in contact with the floor most of the time to reduce potentially injurious stresses on the body. The center of gravity of the body, however, rises and falls almost as much as it does during HIA, thus avoiding prolonged knee flexion.[10] This raising and lowering of the center of gravity, by extending the hip, knee, and ankle joints without actually leaving the floor, requires *work*, the expenditure of energy. This provides for a relatively high exercise intensity.

Athletes have used the plyometric technique for many years, in sports such as track and skiing, to increase power in a workout. These athletes have used plyometric techniques to increase their springing or bounding abilities. For example, picture yourself engaged in either sport and landing and recovering after a forceful jump. The lifting and springing action is called plyometric. You are force-fully loading the weight as you jump and then have a powerful unloading, or springing out of this move.[11]

Although this is an effective method to increase power, it can be stressful to the musculoskeletal system of the average person. In moderate-impact aerobics the plyometric principle of power in movement will be used, but you will load the weight with much less force by simply bending or flexing the knees and the hips, then springing out of this position. This will allow you to increase the intensity safely and also increase power in your leg and hip muscles safely.

> *The sum total of all the stresses on the various vulnerable parts of the body is what determines whether injury occurs.*

In many LIA routines the emphasis is placed on flexing the knees, lowering and then raising the body to an erect position. This can be stressful to the knees of some participants. In addition, many beginners have found that this *down-up* movement is unnatural and requires a great deal of concentration. If the amount of knee flexion is decreased and *emphasis is placed on extending the knees and ankle joints without the feet actually leaving the floor —* as in moderate-impact aerobics — the center of gravity can be raised and lowered effectively. The physiological cost is high, but the bouncy motions are comfortable and stimulating for many participants.[12]

To clarify the differences between the three distinct methods of impact, an example of *stepping-in-place* is:

● *High-impact aerobics:* jogging — both feet off the ground briefly.

● *Low-impact aerobics:* marching — one foot always in contact with the floor.

● *Moderate-impact aerobics:* plyometric techniques using the lift-and-spring action depicted in Figure 7.5.

FIGURE 7.5   Plyometric Technique

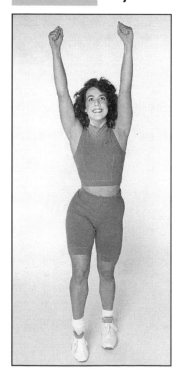

Keeping your R foot flat on the floor, raise your L foot until the tip of your L toe is just barely in contact with the floor. Now alternate the position of the feet to the same tempo that you used for the two previous movements. Lift your body as high as possible as you shift your weight from foot to foot by using the full range of motion of your ankle joints and moderate amounts of knee flexion and extension. Make certain that the heel of the supporting foot is pressed to the floor to maintain a good range of motion of the ankle joint.

The main difference between high-impact jogging and the moderate-impact version is the *rate at which the force is increased on the foot.* Even though the final load on the foot for the MIA step is close in magnitude to that for the HIA step, the load increased much more gradually during the MIA step.

Researchers believe that when high levels of force are exerted on the feet suddenly, the human body is vulnerable to injury. The body is equipped with reflex mechanisms that can control muscle contractions to protect it from mechanical stress. Damage can occur, however, if the forces reach high levels before the reflex mechanisms can provide protection. In practical terms, the springlike motions of MIA are less jarring than the high-impact versions because the body is raised and lowered with control. In HIA, the body is under less control as it falls freely, colliding suddenly with the floor.[13]

Guidelines for using moderate-impact aerobics are as follows:

1. Begin movements by lifting your body upward, rising onto the balls of your feet. Complete each step, whenever possible, by lowering your heels and pressing them gently against the floor. This action produces the springlike motion characteristic of MIA steps. The lifting and lowering of the center of gravity is what increases exercise intensity.

2. Concentrate on leaving at least one foot on the floor most of the time. The purpose of MIA is to reduce the magnitude of impact. Steps such as MIA jogs, jumps, and twists are performed with both feet on the floor, either bearing the weight on both feet, as in a jump, or bearing it on one foot with the second foot lightly touching the floor, as in a twisting step.

   MIA steps that require lifting one foot off the floor, such as kicks and knee-lifts, must be timed carefully so the airborne foot is back on the floor before the opposite foot leaves the floor.

3. Exercise intensity can be increased by traveling directionally across the floor and using the arms through a wide range of movement.

4. To adapt your present LIA or HIA moves to MIA, concentrate on taking the movement up and down while keeping one foot on the floor most of the time. (Not all LIA and HIA steps can be modified to suit MIA. Practice and common sense will help you determine which steps can be adjusted best.) Examples of steps that adapt well to MIA are heel-jacks, jogs, jumps, kicks, knee-lifts, ponies, step-touches, and twists.

5. For variety, mix MIA with LIA and HIA steps.

6. Because the ankle joint is used through a wider range of motion with MIA than with HIA and LIA, it is particularly important to strengthen the tibialis anterior (shin area) and stretch the gastrocnemius and soleus (back lower leg area) muscles during warm-up and cool-down. These precautions will help prevent tightness of the calf as well as muscle imbalance.[14]

CALORIC EXPENDITURE FROM AEROBICS

Research has indicated that, if all of the variables are attended to and duplicated carefully, aerobics can cause substantial energy expenditure of more than *12 calories per minute, with no significant difference in caloric expenditure between low- and high-impact routines* (if these routines are duplicated in style, content, and energy level).[15] This study was carried out using certified instructors (IDEA Foundation and AFAA) and involved two 11-minute sequences of high-impact and low-impact aerobics at a tempo of 148 bpm. For those concerned with weight management, it is exciting to conclude that one can engage in high- or low-impact moves and still expend significant energy and burn calories.

Because the average peak force of LIA can result in impact forces of approximately 1½ times your weight and HIA can result in foot impact approximately 3 times your weight,[16] the impact you choose can be important — especially if you have physical limitations (e.g., obesity, pregnancy, susceptibility to joint injury). Choice of impact, therefore, does not have to be made in regard to caloric expenditure.

AEROBICS TECHNIQUES

The aerobics segment of your fitness hour can be subdivided into six parts, each focusing on the impact in relation to the heart rate intensity you are building, sustaining, or lowering and according to which phase of the hour you are in.

These six parts are:

1. Low-impact aerobics warm-up
2. Power low-impact aerobics
3. High/low-impact aerobics
4. Power low-impact aerobics
5. Low impact aerobics cool-down
6. Post-aerobics stretching

Low-Impact Aerobics Warm-Up

The LIA warm-up consists of simple, low-intensity moves that increase the heart rate gradually. They start with the legs down low and arms below heart level. To increase the intensity gradually, the range of motion of each movement is first increased, and then the use of air and floor space is widened. For example: Step-touch in place with hand claps, punching, or arms shoulder high (Figure 7.6) with hands pointing in (a), and then both hands and toe-touch extending far out, to the side (b). Progress to a grapevine (Figure 7.7), using large arm reaches, then the other low-impact moves (Figures 7.8-7.16). The timeframe is 5 minutes.

FIGURE 7.6 Step Touch

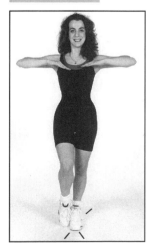

(a) In.

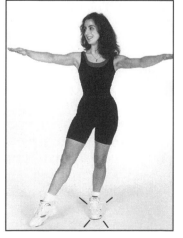

(b) Out.

FIGURE 7.7 Grapevine

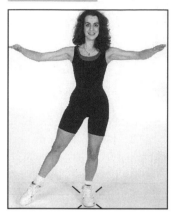

(a)
Step to R side, arms out shoulder high.

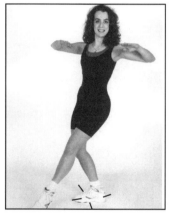

(b)
Step back L, and bring arms in, still shoulder high.

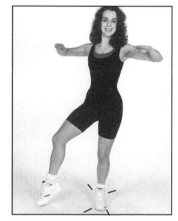

(c)
Step R side.

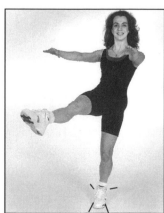

(d)
Weight still R, kick L, arms forward and parallel.

OPTIONS:

Instead of kick,

- touch;
- knee-lift;
- lift-touch forward or backward.

Low-Impact Aerobics Warm-Up

FIGURE 7.8   Bounce 'n Hitch-Kick

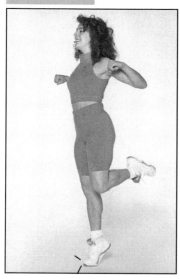

(a)
One-foot bounce while bending other knee, with lower leg pointing back. (1 count)

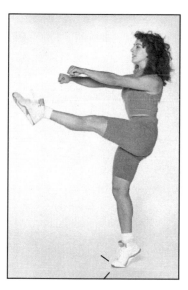

(b)
One-foot bounce and kick same leg forward, waist-high or lower. (1 count)

Low-impact aerobics require that one foot is always in contact with the floor.

FIGURE 7.9   Bounce 'n Tap Series

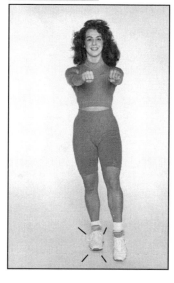

(a)
One-foot bounce on L foot, pointing and tapping R toe forward. Arms punch parallel forward. (1–4 counts)

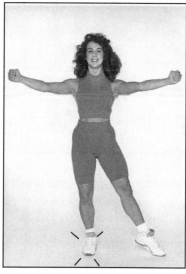

(b)
Weight remains on L foot; bouncing; R toe is now pointing and tapping wide R. Arms follow, wide to sides, palms/fists up. (1–4 counts)

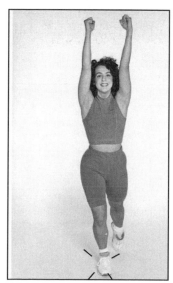

(c)
Weight remains on L bouncing; R toe, is pointing and tapping backward. Arms raise overhead, thumbs back. (1–4 counts)

Next: Alternate by bringing pointing and tapping foot in, and two-foot bounce in place. (1–4 counts)

Shift weight to R foot and repeat series.

Low-Impact Aerobics Warm-Up

FIGURE 7.10 **Heel-Toe Bounce Series**

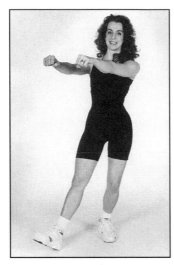

(a)
Bounce R foot while L heel extends forward. Arms forward.
(1 count)

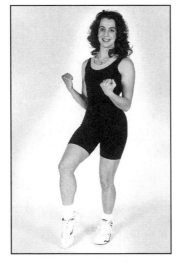

(b)
Bounce R foot, while L toe taps in close. Draw arms in to chest.
(1 count)

Repeat heel out, followed by feet back in together in a transitional move.
(2 counts)

FIGURE 7.11 **Kicks**

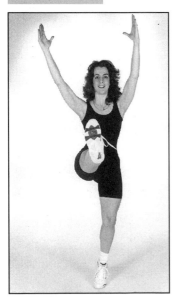

Weight on one foot, kick other leg to only a 90° waist-high level (or lower). Forward or sideward.
(1 count)

OPTIONS:
Add bounce.
(2 counts)

FIGURE 7.12 **Hoe-Down**

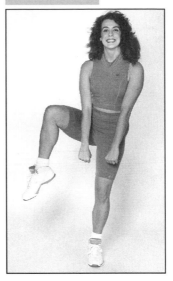

(a)
Bounce R foot, lifting L knee to L side. Arms parallel, punch down.
(1–2 counts)

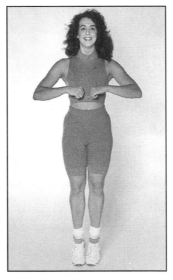

(b)
Feet together bouncing, lift arms chest-high in a half upright-row position (transitional move).
(1 count)

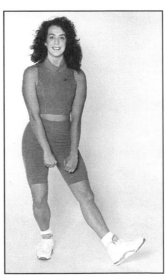

(c)
Bounce L foot, extending R heel forward. Arms parallel, punch down.
(1–2 counts)

Last, repeat (b) transitional move.
(1 count)

Low-Impact Aerobics Warm-Up

FIGURE 7.13 **Knee-Lift Varieties**

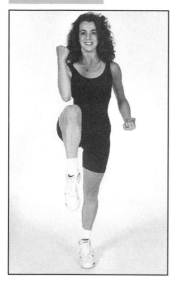

(a)
Step R, knee-lift L knee forward, touch same elbow.
(2 counts)

Reverse.

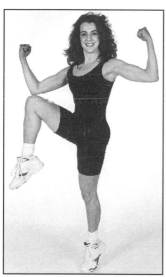

(b)
Step R, knee-lift L knee sideward, same elbow out wide and touch.
(2 counts)

Reverse.

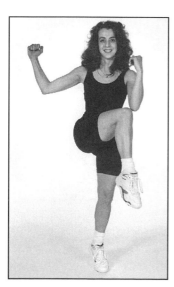

(c)
Step R, knee-lift L knee across body center forward, R (opposite) elbow across chest and touching the knee lifted.
(2 counts)

Reverse.

FIGURE 7.14 **Lunge Side and Bounce**

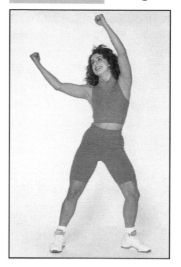

Step and bounce-lunge R, arms overhead, parallel and diagonally high L, head following direction of arms.
(2 counts)

Reverse, shifting weight.
(2 counts)

FIGURE 7.15 **Marching**

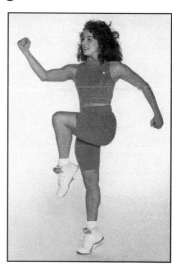

Step-lift, one count each step pattern. Swing arms opposite and big.
(1 count)

FIGURE 7.16 **Side Step-Out**

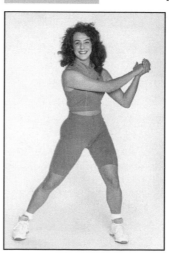

Step out wide stride to R side, bending knees.
(1 count)

Clap hands R.
(1 count)

Reverse.
(2 counts)

Power Low-Impact Aerobics

The moves illustrated increase the load on the large muscles of the legs by bending and extending more, with the accent on lifting or raising the center of gravity while keeping at least one foot firmly on the floor and recovering with an ankle-flexion springing movement. Traveling through space is characteristic with these movements, which really challenge the leg muscles. The examples in Figures 7.17–7.23 are strong low-impact with plyometrics. The timeframe is approximately 10 minutes.

FIGURE 7.19 Fitness Power Walk

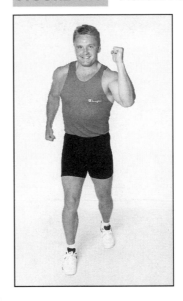

Walk with force, using short-lever or long-lever arms.

FIGURE 7.17 Bouncing and Reaching — Side

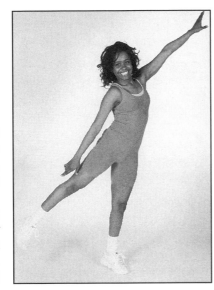

Reach R, extend R arm high, weight on R foot. (1 count)

Bring feet together, arms into center and two-foot bounce. (1 count)

FIGURE 7.20 Two-Foot Jump

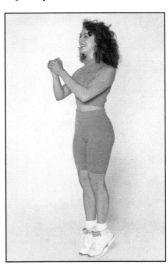

(a) Lift high on balls of feet, without leaving floor. (1 count)

FIGURE 7.18 Bouncing and Reaching — Center

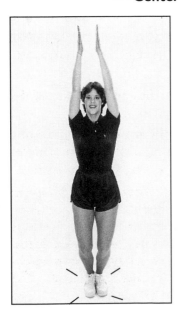

Two-foot bounce and reach high above you. (2 counts)

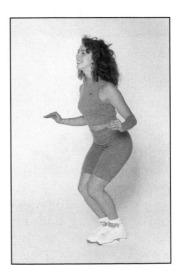

(b) Land and gently press the heels into the floor. (1 count)

Power Low-Impact Aerobics

| FIGURE 7.21   Knee Lift | FIGURE 7.22   Squats | FIGURE 7.23   Twist |

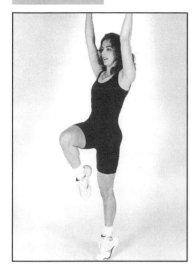

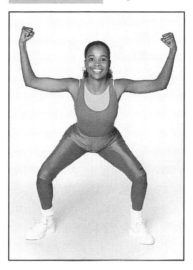

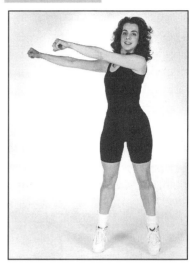

Lift knee while rising to ball of foot. (1 count)

Lower heel of support foot as lifted foot returns to ground. (1 count)

Arms forcefully assist in raising entire body, reaching above shoulder level.

With feet in a wide base of support, toes out, bend knees and hips, and "sit"; curl arms wide and shoulder high, and in. (1 count)

Extend arms out, legs upward to full extension. (1 count)

Shift weight from ball of foot to ball of other foot as you lift your body and twist from side to side. (2 counts)

Note: **You can also easily use these moves as moderate-impact plyometric moves: lunges, jumps, kicks, step-touches, jogs, heel-jacks, ponies.**[16]

High/Low-Impact Aerobics

Here you'll intersperse high-impact moves, in which both feet may leave the floor momentarily, with low-impact moves, in which one foot always remains on the floor. You'll raise your arms overhead more frequently, and raise the knees and feet up higher.

A key point in this segment is that the intensity of the moves you choose must remain high so the heart rate maintains the high, but safe, training zone you've established for cardiorespiratory improvement. *Not more than four high-impact repetitions are performed on the same leg at one time.* Examples are: two high-impact jacks in the wide-stride-and-together leg and arm positions (Figure 7.33), followed by four low-impact power-walking moves with forceful arms (Figure 7.19).

Most *high-impact* moves can be converted easily to *low-impact* moves simply by removing the five basic high-impact movements outlined in Table 7.1. Instead of a take-off and landing, those moves are changed to moves:

● in which one foot remains on the floor as the free foot uses floor and air space; or

● keeping both feet on the ground, incorporating the lifting and lowering plyometric principles described earlier.

To change *low-impact* moves to *high-impact* moves, you simply replace the stationary-foot move and incorporate the high-impact locomotor moves of take-offs and landings (hops, hitch-kicks, leaps, rocks, hop astride, two-foot jumps, or hopscotch-type moves replace a low-impact step move). The timeframe is approximately 15 minutes.

High/Low-Impact Aerobics

TABLE 7.1	Basic High-Impact Locomotor Movements[17]		
Take-Off	**Landing**	**Example**	**Figure**
One foot	same foot	hop; hitch-kick	7.24; 7.25
One foot	opposite foot	leap; rock	7.26; 7.27-7.29
One foot	two feet	astride	7.30
Two feet	two feet	jump (widestride or together)	7.31-7.33
Two feet	one foot	hopscotch; polka	7.34-7.35

Source: *Aerobic Dance — A Way to Fitness*, 2d edition, by Karen S. Mazzeo et al (Englewood, CO: Morton Publishing, 1987), p. 112.

FIGURE 7.24 Hops — Single and Double

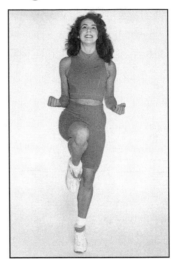

Single Hops: Hop R, forward lifting L knee. (1 count)

Double Hops: Repeat R hop. (2 counts)

FIGURE 7.25 Hitch-Kick

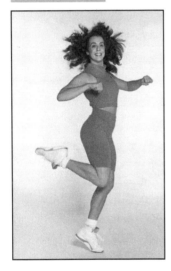

(a) Hop on L as R foot lifts back, knee bent.

OPTIONS:

Pull arms back forcefully. (1 count)

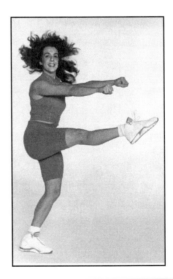

(b) Hop L again, kicking R forward, waist-high or lower.

OPTIONS:

Arms forcefully parallel, punching forward. (1 count)

Reverse. (2 counts)

FIGURE 7.26 Leap

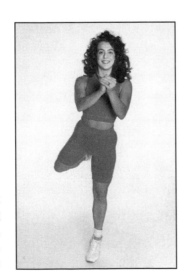

With weight L (not shown) take off, propelling body forward and upward, landing on R foot. (4 counts)

FIGURE 7.27 Rock Side-To-Side

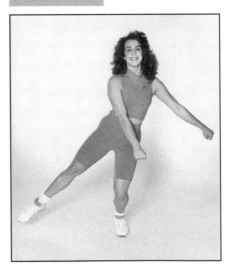

Hop on R foot to R side, placing weight over R leg (knee and ankle flexed), lifting L leg out to side. (1 count)

Reverse.

High/Low-Impact Aerobics

FIGURE 7.28 **Rock Forward**

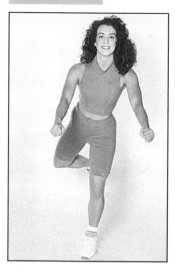

Rock (hop) R into forward lean, lifting L leg back and up for balance.
(1 count)

FIGURE 7.29 **Rock Backward**

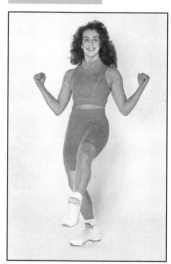

Rock (hop) L backward into backward lean, lifting R leg forward and up for balance.
(1 count)

FIGURE 7.30 **Astride**

With weight R or L (not shown), hop to astride or straddle position, loading weight onto both feet by bending knees.
(1 count)

(Usually preceded by or followed with another move.)

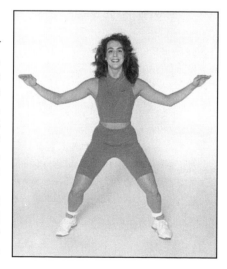

Two-Foot Jump

FIGURE 7.31 **Lunge**

Two-foot scissors jump forward on R foot, bending R while keeping L leg extended back (still bearing weight on L) in wide forward/backward lunge position, L arm forward, R arm back. (1 count)

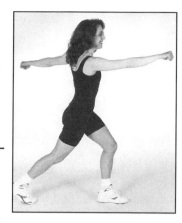

OPTIONS:

(1) Jump back to two-feet together and center (1 count), then reverse the forward and backward legs and arms, lunging and jumping back to center. (2 counts)

(2) Reverse directly from forward/backward lunge, (1 count), to opposite forward/backward lunge position. (1 count)

FIGURE 7.32 **Jumps — Feet Together**

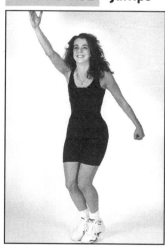

(a)
Jump sideward, forward, or back. Hold.
(2 counts)

Reverse.

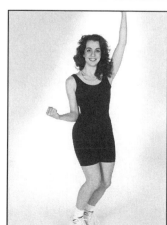

OPTIONS:

(b)
Use skiing arms position with L elbow close, R elbow high and wide, when jumping R. Reverse arms when you reverse feet.

High/Low-Impact Aerobics

FIGURE 7.33 **Jumping Jacks**

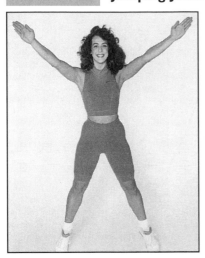

(a)

(b)

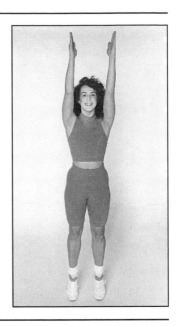

When executing two-foot jump to side in *wide-stride position*, followed by two-foot jump *together*, this becomes a jumping jack. Arms can work wide and together with legs, or in opposition (not shown).

OPTIONS:

Coordination Pattern: Jump wide (a); together with high arms (b); jump wide (a); together with low arms (not shown). (4 counts)

FIGURE 7.34 **Hopscotch —**

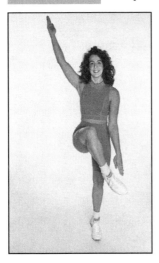

Forward (a)
Hop to astride position (Figure 7.30) and with weight on R foot, hop and touch L foot raised forward to lowered R hand (a knee-open position). (2 counts)
For balance, reach L hand diagonally skyward, thumb back. Reverse.

Back (b)
Hop to stride position (Figure 7.30), and with weight on L foot, hop and touch R foot raised backward to lowered L hand. (2 counts)
For balance, reach R hand diagonally skyward, thumb back. Reverse.

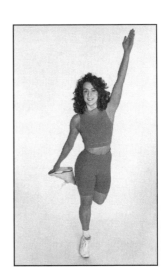

NOTE:

If you have sensitive (injury-prone or recent surgery) knees, avoid this exercise variety.

FIGURE 7.35 **Polka**

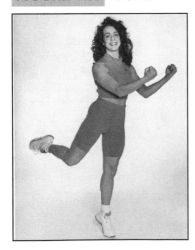

Many popular social dances, or dance steps and gestures, are aerobics possibilities.[18]

(a)
Hop R, lifting L leg backward.
(1 count)

(b)
Step L, in close quickly.
(1/2 count)
Step R, in close quickly.
(1/2 count)
Step L, in close quickly.
(1/2 count)

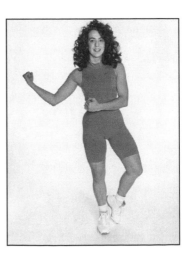

AEROBICS VARIETY: FUNK MOVES

Funk aerobics are exercise moves developed from the culturally rich areas of jazz dance, ballet, street dance, gymnastics floor-exercise competition, and other rhythmical forms of aesthetic, emotionally expressive movement.

Funk aerobics include numerous expressive trunk, elbow and knee moves (Figure 7.36), funk walking (Figure 7.37) that mimics movie and television characters, and animation moves such as Roger Rabbit and funky chicken.

Creative expression and attitude prevail in funk exercise movement. Body gestures include the extremely big and wide-open positions (Figure 7.38), followed quickly by closed, tight, head gesture or hair-tossing moves (Figure 7.39). The only limitation for funk aerobics lies in your own resources, experience, and individual creativity — which for all of us are unlimited!

For yet another creative option, *combine your favorite aerobics moves with the step bench* (Chapter 8). "Step Training the Funky Cha-Cha" and other dance moves opens up the possibility for unlimited program variety.

FIGURE 7.36

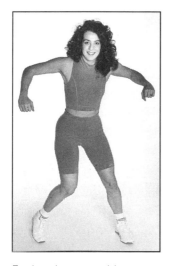

Funky ebows and knees.

FIGURE 7.37

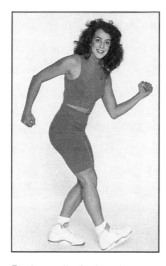

Funky walks/animation.

FIGURE 7.38

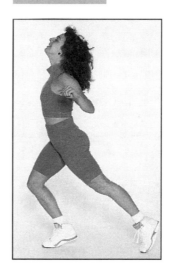

Funky open position.

FIGURE 7.39

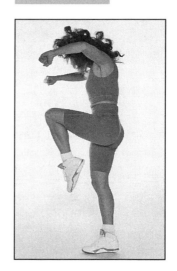

Funky closed position.

Power Low-Impact Aerobics

Again, power LIA consists of the center-of-gravity lifting, hip-knee-ankle extending moves, followed by the knee-flexion, ankle springing-action moves in which one foot is always in contact with the floor, to keep the force of impact low (Figures 7.17-7.24). The timeframe is approximately 5 minutes.

Low-Impact Aerobics Cool-Down

These are the lower intensity moves needed to lower your heart rate gradually. They are still active and rhythmic, using a full range of motion, but now are low-level and slower, half-the-tempo moves. They are the same as those used in the warm-up, Figures 7.6-7.16. The timeframe is approximately 10 minutes.

Post-Aerobics Stretching

Stretching the lower-body muscles to aid blood returning to the heart and preventing blood pooling in the legs is performed by standing static stretches for the hamstrings (Figure 6.11), quadriceps/iliopsoas (Figure 6.13), and calf muscles (Figure 6.12). The timeframe can be approximately 3–5 minutes.

AEROBICS GESTURE, STEP, AND PATTERN CUES

You now can easily follow the instructor-choreographed moves during class, or design an individualized program for yourself, according to your favorite moves and combinations. A list of gesture, step, and pattern cues follows, to assist with your program planning. Having the knowledge provides the freedom to choose and goal-set.

- **Arm Circle:** Circle-back; forward; big; small.
- **Bounce, Hitch-Kick:** One-foot bounce, kick; other-foot bounce, kick. (Figure 7.8)
- **Bounce 'n Tap Pattern:** Forward, side, back, together (or hold); forward, side, back, together (or hold). (Figures 7.9, 7.12b)
- **Bounce 'n Tap Sequences:** Right forward 4, side 4, back 4, hold 4; repeat left forward 4, etc. Right forward 3 and hold 1, side 3 and hold 1, back 3 and hold 1, hold 4; repeat left forward 3 and hold 1, etc. Right forward 2, side 2, back 2, hold 2; repeat left forward 2, etc. Right forward, side, back, hold; left forward, side, back, hold. (Figures 7.9, 7.12b)
- **Bounce, Two Feet:** Bounce. Or: Lift, bounce. (Figure 7.12b)
- **Bounce, Two Feet Variation:** Punch, bounce.
- **Bounce-Step, Bounce-Touch:** Two-foot bounce-step, one foot bounce & touch; two-foot bounce-step, one foot bounce & touch. (Figures 7.12b, 7.9b)
- **Bounce Steps, with Side Touch:** One foot bounce, touch, one foot bounce, touch.
- **Cha-Cha:** Cross (right forward), (left step) back, step-step, step; cross (left forward), (right step) back, step-step, step.
- **Cha-Cha, with Kick Pattern:** Cross, back, step, kick, step, step, step-step, step.
- **Charleston Flapper Walk:** Step and swing forward, step and swing back.
- **Cross-Step Forward, Touch to Side:** Cross, touch; cross, touch.
- **Cross-Step, Hop:** Cross, hop; cross, hop.
- **"Doubles" Knees and Kicks:** Knee-lift, down, up, down; kick, down, up, down. (Figures 7.13, 7.11)
- **Double Hops:** Hop, hop and punch; hop, hop and punch.
- **Double Hop, Hitch Kick:** Hop, hop-kick; hop, hop-kick.
- **Fall Back 'n Jump Forward Pattern:** Hop, step-step, rock-back, rock-forward. (Figures 7.35, 7.29, 7.28)
- **Funk:**
  Elbows and Knees: Bend/extend/wide/out, relax; repeat left. (Figure 7.36)
  Walks and Animation: Attitude walkin', walkin'. (Figure 7.37)

- **Open and Closed:** Strut wide, in, wide, in (Figures 7.38, 7.39), and reverse.
- **Gallop:** Step, slide and lift.
- **Grapevine:** Side, back, side, touch; side, back, side, touch. (Figure 7.7)
- **Grapevine Varieties:**
  'n Kick: Side, back, side, kick. (Figure 7.7)
  'n Hop: Side, back, side, hop-clap (or hop-click, or hop-punch).
  'n Jump-Clap: Side, back, side, jump-clap.
- **Heel-Out, Toe-in Bounce Pattern:** Out, in, out, bounce; out, in, out, bounce. (Figures 7.10, 7.12)
- **Hip Thrust:** Astride, thrust; astride, thrust.
- **Hoe-down:** Bounce/lift, punch down; two-foot bounce; bounce/heel touch; two-foot bounce. (Figure 7.12)
- **Hops, Single:** Hop/lift; repeat left. **Double:** Hop, hop (same foot). (Figure 7.24)
- **Hop, Hitch-Kick:** Hop, hop-kick (or Kick-back, forward). (Figure 7.25)
- **Hop, Kick:** Hop, kick; hop, kick. (Figures 7.24, 7.11); reverse.
- **Hopscotch:** Astride, hop, astride, hop. (Figures 7.30, 7.24)
- **Hopscotch, Variety:** Astride, hop-touch; astride, hop-touch. (Figures 7.30, 7.34)
- **Hustle:** Jog, jog, jog, lift-clap; jog-back, jog, jog, lift-clap.
  Cross-Elbow Touch: Jog, jog, jog, elbow-touch; jog, jog, jog, elbow-touch.
  High Impact: Hop, hop, hop, lift; hop, hop, hop, lift.
  Low Impact: Pace-walk, walk, walk, lift; pace-walk-back, walk, walk, lift.
- **Jazz Touch — Out 'n In pattern:** Out, in, out, shift-your-weight; out, in, out, weight-right. (Figure 7.6)
- **Jazz Touch — Forward 'n Backward Pattern:** Forward, back, forward, shift-your-weight; forward, back, forward, weight-right.
- **Jog:** Jog — heel first.
  Circling: Jog, 2, 3, 4, 5, 6, 7, 8. Jog — left, 2, 3, 4, 5, 6, 7, 8.
- **Jumps:**
  Big/Little: Big, turn-clap, little and clap; turn-clap, little-clap; turn-clap, little-clap; turn-front-clap, little-clap.
  One-Foot Jump: Jump-right; jump-left.
  Two-Foot Jump: Jump and clap! (Figure 7.20)
  Circling: 3 o'clock, 6 o'clock, 9 o'clock, noon; reverse-and-9 o'clock, 6 o'clock, 3 o'clock, 12 o'clock.
  Forward 'n Backward: Jump-forward, jump-back.
  'n Land, Widestride: Jump and land-wide, hold. (Figure 7.33)
  Side Jump, Clap: Jump-side, clap; side, clap. (Figure 7.32a)

Ski Jump: Jump-side, hold; jump-side, hold. (Figure 7.32b)

● **Jumping Jacks:**

Regular: Stride-clap, together-slap.

Coordinated: Astride-wide, together-clap. (Figure 7.33)

Crazy: Stride, cross; stride, cross.

Double Pattern: X, high I, X, low I. (Figure 7.33)

● **Kicks:** Kick right; repeat left. Or, Kick, bounce, kick, bounce. (Figure 7.11)

● **Knee-Lift:** Power lift, power lower; repeat left. (Figure 7.21)

● **Knee-Lift Elbow-Touch, Varieties:**

Same Side: Step-lift, elbow-touch-same; repeat left. (Figure 7.13a)

Open to Side: Step-lift, elbow-touch-open; repeat left. (Figure 7.13b)

Crossed: Step-lift, cross-elbow-touch; repeat left. (Figure 7.13c)

High Intensity: Hop-lift, elbow-touch-(same/open/crossed).

● **Leap:** Push-off, leap forward, and clap; repeat left. (Figure 7.26)

● **Lunges:**

Forward: Forward lunge, 2, 3, 4, 5, 6, 7, 8; walk-through-and-lunge, 2, 3, 4, 5, 6, 7, 8.

Scissor: Jump-forward, scissor-jump. (Figure 7.31)

Side: Lunge-side and bounce (the holding counts). (Figure 7.14)

Side, with Arm Circling: Lunge-3 o'clock, hold; 6 o'clock, hold; 9 o'clock, hold; noon, hold; reverse counterclockwise.

Side-Bounce 'n Sway: Lunge-side and bounce; sway-lunge and bounce. (Figure 7.14)

● **March:** Left, right; forward, to-the-rear, side. (Figure 7.15)

● **Polka:** Hop-step, step-step; hop-step, step-step. (Figure 7.35)

Circling: To-the-right, back, side, forward.

Low-Impact: Step, step, step, hold; step, step, step, hold.

Side-to-Side: To-the-left; to-the-right.

● **Prance:** March, hop-lift march, hop-lift march. (Figure 7.15 with a hop.)

● **Quads 'n Hams Coordination Pattern:** Step, lift-front, step, lift-back. (Figure 7.34)

Variety: Step, lift-front left, step, lift-front right; step, lift-back left, step, lift-back right. (Figures 7.30, 7.34)

● **Reach:** Bounce-step, reach; bounce-step, reach. (Figures 7.17 and 7.18)

● **Rock:**

Big, Forward 'n Backward: Rock-forward and back. (Figures 7.28 and 7.29)

Side-to-Side: Rock-side; side. (Figure 7.27)

Side-to-Side Variety: Rock-side and punch; side and punch.

● **Shake Up, Shake Down:** Shake, two, three, four; shake-down, six, seven, eight.

● **Side Coordination Pattern:** Side (right), together (left), side (right), touch (left); side (left), together (right), side (left), touch (right).

● **Side Step-Out:** Side, clap; side clap. (Figure 7.16)

● **Skip:** Step, hop; step, hop. (Figure 7.24)

● **Slides:** Step, together-step.

● **Slide, Bend, Jump, Clap Pattern:** Slide, bend, jump, clap; slide, bend, jump, clap.

● **Squats:** Sit, extend. (Figure 7.22)

● **Step, Hop:** Step, hop (Figure 7.24)

Circling: Step, hop to the side; step, hop to the back; step, hop to the side; step, hop front.

● **Step, Hop, Step, Kick Pattern:** Step (right), hop (right), step (left), kick (right).

● **Step, Kick:** Step, kick; step, kick.

Circling: Step, kick; two; three; four; five; six; seven; eight.

'n Punch-Down: Step, kick-side and punch down, step, kick-front, and punch down.

Sidekick: Step, side-kick and click; step, side-kick and click.

● **Step, Lift, Touch, Lift Pattern:** Step (right), lift (left), touch (left), lift (left); step (left), lift (right), touch (right), lift (right).

● **Stride 'n Twist Pattern:** Stride, cross, turn, hold, lift, touch, kick, touch.

● **The Twist:** Step forward and twist-down, 2, 3, 4; twist-up, 2, 3, 4; walk-through-forward (or back) and twist, 2, 3, 4; twist-up, 2, 3, 4.

Power Twist: Lift and twist, down; lift and twist, down. (Figure 7.23)

● **Walk:** Power-walk-forward and (count each pace walk). (Figure 7.19)

● **Walk Varieties, with Creative Arm Gestures:**

Backward: Pace-walk back and (count).

Diagonally: Pace-walk diagonally-right, and (count).

Sideward: Pace-walk-side, and (count).

● **Widestrides:**

Arm Crossover: Stride-bend and cross, up, raise, out and down.

● **New gestures, steps, and patterns presented in class:**

●

●

●

●

●

●

Goal Setting Challenge

Set a goal that challenges your ability to master the moves and develop sequences and then entire routines. You can do it!

Developing Goal Scripts for Chapter 7

DIRECTIONS: Write complete sentences for each segment below. Combine your responses to all four segments. This goal script is designed around your needs and choices. Read it (or make an audiotape and play it) twice daily, morning and evening, until you master it.

❶ State one goal in positive, *present-tense* language. Ask yourself, "What will I experience — see, hear, taste, smell, feel — in regard to the results? Keep in mind that all powerful goals use the SMART formula: specific, measurable, achievable, realistic, timely.

_____

_____

❷ State your *pleasure-value reasons*. Ask yourself, "Why am I totally committed to achieving this goal? What am I choosing to feel?"

_____

_____

❸ State your *pain-avoidance value reasons*. Ask yourself, "What painful values do I choose to avoid feeling?"

_____

_____

❹ State *immediate action(s)* you can take in the next 24 hours. Use positive, present-tense verbs such as *choose* and verbs ending with "ing."

_____

_____

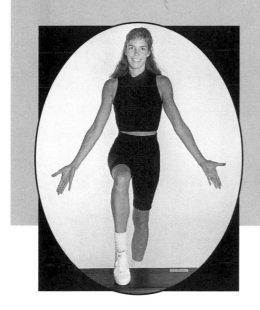

Aerobic Exercise:
Step Training (Option 2)

Motivation to stay with any fitness program will be enhanced by adding variety to your program when you need a change. Two unique possibilities to add to the aerobic segment of your program are (a) bench/step training, and (b) aerobic intervals of bench/step training with strength training, involving the bench/step and resistance tubing.

PRINCIPLES OF BENCH/STEP TRAINING

Bench/step training, or "step training," is sweeping the aerobic exercise and fitness industry with a new burst of enthusiasm. It is the hottest aerobic trend of the 1990s. Because it is a relatively new training modality, all of the related problems and injuries have not yet been fully researched or assessed. The following information and guidelines have been presented by various researchers promoting the activity, and companies promoting products to use with the activity.[1, 2, 3, 4, 5]

Definition and Benefits

Step training is an exercise that involves stepping up and down on a platform or bench with a variety of upper-torso movements added for further challenge. It has a variety of names: bench or step aerobics, bench or step training, bench stepping, and stepping, to name just a few. All refer to the same activity.

The benefits are many. The main advantage to a step training program is that it is primarily a *high-intensity activity* to promote cardiorespiratory fitness but *with low impact* for safety concerns. A vast majority of the moves can involve one foot supporting your weight, either on the bench platform or on the floor. Other benefits are:

- It is an excellent conditioning workout for the muscles of the legs, hips, and buttocks.
- Upper torso movements provide conditioning for muscles of the arms, shoulders, chest, and back, and therefore a balanced and complete workout that strengthens and tones the entire body. This becomes apparent later if you advance to using 1–4 lb light hand weights in a controlled manner in conjunction with your stepping moves.
- As an effective cardiovascular workout, step training has aerobic benefits equal to running 7 miles per hour (mph), yet has the potentially low-impact equivalence of walking at a 3-mph pace.[6]
- This workout allows class versatility. The basic moves are simple, and by introducing various step patterns, participants at all levels can be challenged simultaneously. Regardless of gender or age, individuals can work at their own fitness level simply by doing fewer (or more) arm gestures, by adjusting the height of the bench, and by adding or omitting hand weights.

Choosing Your Bench Height

When selecting a bench height, consider the following factors:

- As a beginner or novice who has not exercised regularly, or has limited coordination, or no experience in step training, you initially should select a 4" to 6" bench. For the 12" bench shown in the chapter opening photo, this represents the basic 4" platform, and at most one 2" support block on each end.

- As an intermediate or regular step trainer with a "physically fit" level of cardiorespiratory fitness, choose an 8"–10" step. An 8" bench equals a 4" platform (shown in the chapter opening) and two 2" support blocks. For a 10" bench, add three 2" support blocks.

- Advanced or skilled regular step trainers with a high level of cardiovascular fitness should choose a 10"–12" step (a 4" platform plus a maximum of 4 support blocks on each end).

- Taller individuals may prefer a bench step of 8"–12".

- Regardless of level of fitness or experience, you should not select a step height that allows the knee to flex less than 90° (Figure 8.1) when the knee is weight-bearing. *If your knees advance beyond your toes as you step up, the platform is too high.*

An optional test for bench height is shown in Figure 8.2. Place one foot flat on top of the bench; allow a 3" drop from hip to knee for safe movement up to the top of the bench.

Body Alignment and Stepping Technique

Good posture is required for a safe, injury-free workout. Proper alignment and stepping technique are:

- Keep your back straight, head and chest up, shoulders back, abdomen tight, and buttocks tucked under hips, with eyes on the platform (Figure 8.3).

- As much as possible, keep your shoulders aligned over your hips. Lean forward with the whole body. Don't bend from the hips or round the shoulders and lean forward or backward.

- Step up lightly, making sure the whole foot lands on the platform, with the heel bearing your weight.

FIGURE 8.1

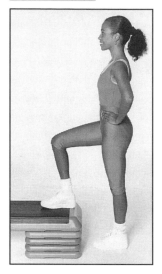

Knee position indicating correct height for bench.

FIGURE 8.2

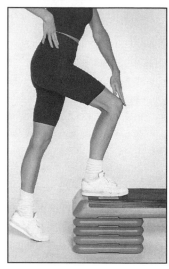

Optional test for bench height, allowing 3" drop from hip to knee.

- At the top, straighten your legs but don't lock your knees; keep them "soft."

- As you step down, stay close to the platform. (Figure 8.4) Land on the ball of the foot, then bring the heel down onto the floor, before taking the next step.

FIGURE 8.3

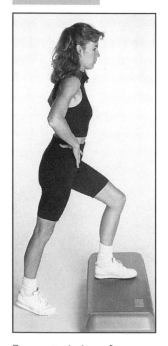

Proper technique for stepping up.

FIGURE 8.4

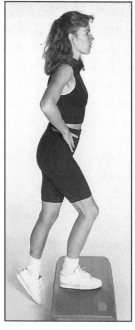

Proper technique for stepping down.

Step Training Postures

Three common step training errors to avoid are illustrated in Figures 8.5, 8.7, and 8.9. The man is demonstrating incorrect postural techn... exercise. In Figures 8.6, 8.8, and 8.10, performing correctly.[7]

Incorrect Hip/Leg Extension

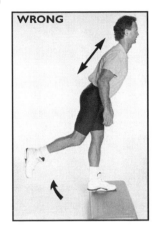

Undesirable curve of lower back with excessive rear leg lift and forward body lean.

Correct Position for Leg Extension

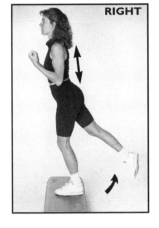

Stand tall on platform and extend the rear lifting leg *back* not up.

Incorrect Side Step-Out Squats

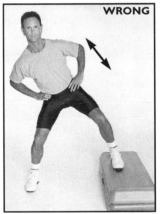

Tendency to lean too far out to the side, which places too much stress on the knee.

Correct Position for Step-Out Squats

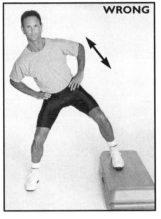

Balance your weight evenly, keeping center of gravity squarely within your legs.

Incorrect Step-Back Lunges From Platform

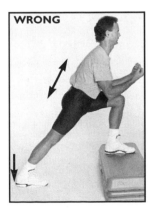
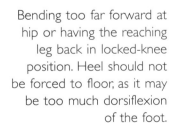

Bending too far forward at hip or having the reaching leg back in locked-knee position. Heel should not be forced to floor, as it may be too much dorsiflexion of the foot.

Correct Position for Step-Back Lunges From Platform

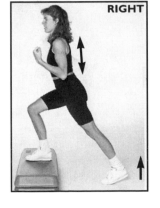

Keep body weight predominantly over platform leg, and knee over toes. Leg reaching back should make floor contact with knee slightly flexed. This reduces chance for joint trauma. Back heel is raised off the floor.

Stepping to Music

Music plays a significant role, providing the underlying structure of a step training program. The tempo of the music (measured as beats per minute (bpm) determines the speed and develops the progression of the movement performed.

Using music with a bpm of 118–125 is best. This will keep the movements controlled. Advanced workouts that follow all safety guidelines of alignment and technique may include tempos up to 135 bpm.

Listed in Table 8.1 are class segments with the suggested time durations and tempos of each.[8]

TABLE 8.1	Suggested Times and Tempos	
Duration (mins.)	Segment	Beats per Minute
10	1. Warm-Up	130–140
20–40	2. Aerobic Stepping and	118–120
3–5	Aerobic Cool-Down	118–120
10–15	3. Strength Training	120–130
5–10	4. Stretching	<100

Step Technique Progression

Beginners should start on a 4" bench, using no weights, at a moderate tempo for no more than 10 minutes per session. As you progress in skill and fitness level, you can increase the length of time stepping. When you can complete an entire session easily, you can raise the platform height, increase the music tempo, use the arms through a wider range of motion, and add 1-lb to 4-lb hand weights.

Only one variable should be changed per session. Don't increase platform height and add weights at the same time. Increasing several variables at the same time doesn't allow your body time to adapt adequately to these changes and stressors.

Start with your hands on your hips, and concentrate on your feet and legs as your first priority. Once you've become proficient with the basic footwork skills and your fitness level has improved, increase the intensity of your program through your arm movements. This can include complicated arm gestures *or* the use of hand weights.

The arm movements used with or without weights are those taken from the strength training programs that use long- and short-lever moves safely in a full range-of-motion action. *All arm movements*

must move with the step pattern. This means that arms go forward when stepping on the bench, back when stepping off, and up on a propulsion move. Think to use muscle more than momentum (i.e., control), and you will keep it a safer workout.

A few precautions are:

- Avoid excessive arm movements over your head.
- Maintain appropriate speed for safe and effective movement.
- Do not perform more than 8 counts (4 repeaters) on one leg at a time. Repeated foot impact without variation is potentially harmful.
- Do not pivot or twist the knee on the weight-bearing leg.
- Do not step up with your back toward the platform.
- If you are pregnant, check with your doctor before starting a step program. If you are cleared by your doctor, make certain to keep your heart rate at 23 beats or below for a 10-second count. A step height of no more than 6" is recommended during pregnancy.
- If you feel faint or dizzy or if any exercise causes pain or severe discomfort, stop the exercise immediately but continue to move around.
- Maintain muscular balance by working opposing muscle groups equally (e.g., quads/hamstrings).
- Limit one person to a bench at a time.
- For the bench in the opening photo, the maximum is four support blocks on each end of the platform.

ADDING HAND-HELD WEIGHTS TO STEPPING

Using 1-lb to 4-lb hand-held weights in a step-training program allows you to increase both exercise intensity for continual cardiovascular fitness gains and muscular strength and tone, especially in the upper torso (Figure 8.11). The low-impact nature of step training, along with controlled stepping patterns performed at a moderate tempo, allows you to use hand-held weights,[9] provided that you adhere to the following safety precautions and those mentioned previously.

1. Add hand weights, using 1-lb or 2-lb weights, only after you are proficient at step training and

FIGURE 8.11

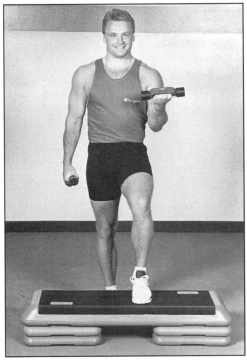

Hand-held weights used in conjunction with step training.

when you have achieved an intermediate level of fitness.

2. Do not use hand weights if you:
   - Have high blood pressure.
   - Have a history of heart disease.
   - Have low-back pain.
   - Have arthritis.
   - Have other chronic or temporary orthopedic problems.
   - Are past the first trimester of pregnancy.
   - Are significantly overweight.

3. When you begin using light weights, use them for just one routine per session, and gradually build up your endurance. Start low and go slow.

4. Begin by using slow, small range of motion with short-lever, nonrotational arm movements, and never use flinging or uncontrolled movements.

5. Do not maintain arms at or above shoulder level for extended periods (i.e., overuse tendons that stabilize the shoulder joint and elevate blood pressure unnecessarily).

6. Avoid full-arm extension moves in short counts of music.

7. Do not use weights while performing propulsion steps.

8. Feel free to put down weights at any time during your workout. Place them safely under the bench or where you'll not step on them accidentally.

ADJUSTING YOUR INTENSITY

To decrease or increase your heart-rate, try the following measures:

To decrease intensity:

1. Do not use weights.
2. Keep hands on hips.
3. Lower bench height.
4. Perform movements only on floor.
5. Decrease music tempo.

To increase intensity:

1. Make larger range-of-motion arm movements.
2. Add 2" support blocks to bench height.
3. Add 1-lb to 4-lb hand-held weights.
4. Increase music tempo.

STEP BENCH USING TUBING

Chapter 10 presents a variety of exercises using tubing in combination with the step bench, for either weight training alone or for an *interval step training/ strength training workout*. The key to the latter workout is incorporating 1-minute intervals of tubing exercises using the bench, with the body pressed into a bent-knees position on the action of the exercise. This position helps to keep the heart rate in the training zone during strength training and provides another safe, unique variety for the aerobic exercise segment of your fitness program.

In sum, incorporating a bench/step training program into your lifetime fitness plan has many advantages and benefits. It is a high-intensity form of exercise that sustains the training zone heart rate needed for the cardiorespiratory training effect to occur. Yet it is low-impact and safe, as one foot remains on the bench or the floor. Safety precautions include selecting the correct bench height, having good body positioning and alignment, introducing variety in technique to prevent overuse, and following the guidelines for incorporating arm gestures. Adding weights and resistance tubing can work together to establish an exciting new variety of aerobic training.

STEP TECHNIQUE

The step training techniques that follow represent movement depicting:

- the warm-up and step aerobics (the strength training and cooling down with the step/bench are presented in Chapters 10 and 11);
- directional approaches and orientations (your body in relation to the bench)
- base steps
- basic step patterns
- variations possible, using base steps and basic step patterns (see Figure 8.12).

These step techniques are photographed and described by the "mirroring technique" for all *front* views shown (actual left of model is your right). Natural photography is used and described for all *side* and *rear* views, including traveling patterns that have a side or rear-view portion. The words and the movements, therefore, are to be performed *exactly* as shown.

If you're following the movements of an instructor, position the bench for maximum visibility.

FIGURE 8.12

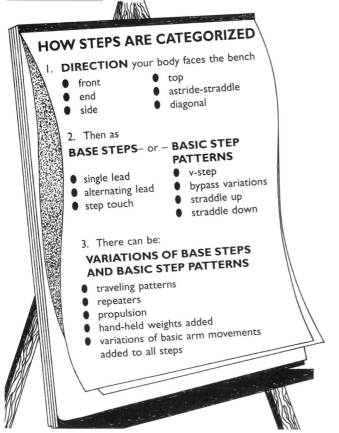

HOW STEPS ARE CATEGORIZED

1. **DIRECTION** your body faces the bench
   - front
   - end
   - side
   - top
   - astride-straddle
   - diagonal

2. Then as
   BASE STEPS– or – **BASIC STEP PATTERNS**
   - single lead
   - alternating lead
   - step touch
   - v-step
   - bypass variations
   - straddle up
   - straddle down

3. There can be:
   VARIATIONS OF BASE STEPS AND BASIC STEP PATTERNS
   - traveling patterns
   - repeaters
   - propulsion
   - hand-held weights added
   - variations of basic arm movements added to all steps

Warm-Up

The warm-up begins with active, low-level, rhythmic, limbering, standing, range-of-motion types of exercises that raise the body's core temperature slightly, initiate muscular movements, and prepare you for more strenuous moves to come. Involve the step-bench by performing moves that integrate the floor and the bench. Example: Perform bench step taps, with bicep curls (Figure 8.13). Use low-impact moves that allow you to adjust to the height and contour of the bench, such as stepping up and down at half the tempo, marching on top of the bench, or straddling the bench and alternating tapping on top of the bench (Figure 8.14). The timeframe is approximately 5 minutes.

FIGURE 8.13

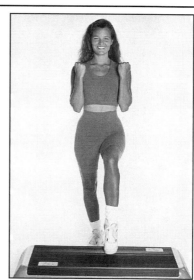

Bench step taps with bicep curls.

FIGURE 8.14

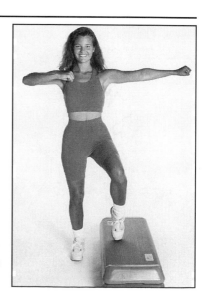

Alternate tapping on top from the straddle position.

After the muscles, tendons, ligaments, and joints are loose and pliable, exercise takes the form of slow, sustained, static stretching. Static stretching, probably the most popular, easiest, and safest form of stretching, involves stretching a muscle or muscle group gradually to the point of limitation, then holding that position for approximately 15 seconds. The stretch is repeated to the opposite side. Several repetitions of each stretch are performed. Static stretching is recommended when muscles are *warm* (after the initial active phase of the warm-up and later after intense physical activity).

Stretch all major muscles from head to toe. Chapter 6 presents ideas with special consideration for the major muscle groups in the legs (the thighs, hips, and calves), as step training is lower body-intensive. When step training, the bench can be used as a fixed object to enhance stretching (Figures 8.15–8-18).[10]

Breathing Technique

Breathe continuously. Your entire system, especially your working muscles, constantly need oxygen. Holding your breath and turning red is never appropriate. While performing the warm-up and cool-down stretching (or any strengthening exercise), exhale when you stretch, by puckering your lips and breathing out, and inhale when you relax your muscles. Cue yourself: "Breathe out and stretch"; "breathe in and relax." The timeframe for the warm-up stretching segment is approximately 5 minutes.

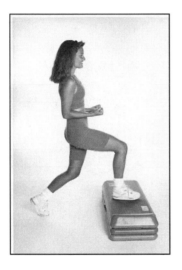

FIGURE 8.15

Hip flexors — facing the bench.

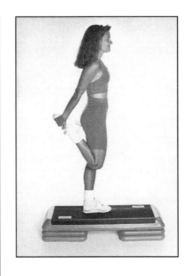

FIGURE 8.16

Quadricep stretch — standing on the bench.

FIGURE 8.17

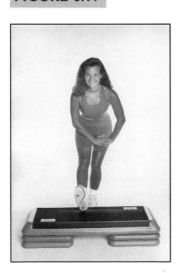

Hamstring stretch — facing the bench.

FIGURE 8.18

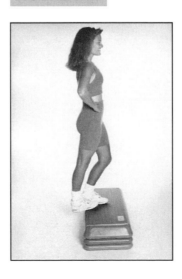

Calf stretch — standing on top of the bench.

Directional Approaches to Bench

Initial movement onto the bench can begin from one of the following directions (the direction your body *faces* the bench):

- front
- end
- side
- top
- astride/ straddle
- diagonal

FIGURE 8.19 From the Front

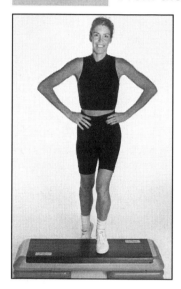

Facing the bench squarely.

FIGURE 8.20 From the End

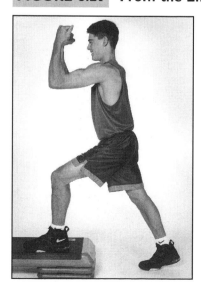

Facing the end of the bench.

FIGURE 8.21 From the Side

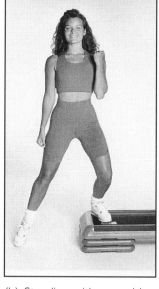 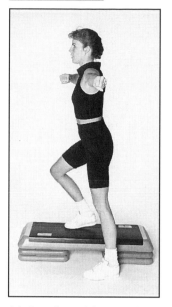

(a) Standing with your side next to the bench's side.

(b) Standing with your side next to the end of the bench.

For both (a) and (b), step up with foot that is closest to the side of the bench.

FIGURE 8.22 From the Top

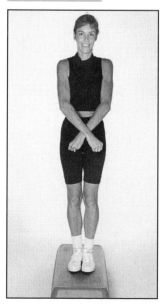 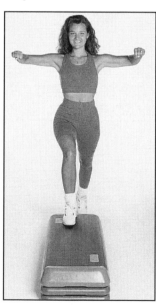

(a) Atop, facing the bench's end, with feet together (shown); or feet in a forward/backward stride.

(b) Atop, standing at the back end of the bench, step off the back in a forward/backward stride.

FIGURE 8.23 Astride / Straddle

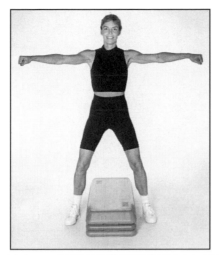

Facing the bench's end, standing astride or straddle position, with bench between your feet.

FIGURE 8.24 From the Diagonal

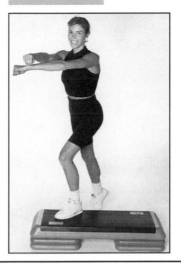

Facing on an angle toward corner when beginning a bypass pattern.

Base Steps

Three base steps may be performed using a variety of directional approaches/orientations. They are identified as:

- a *single* lead step, in which the *same* foot leads *every 4-count cycle*. (Figure 8.25)

- an *alternate* lead step, in which the right and left foot both serve as the lead foot, *alternately initiating every 4 counts*, requiring a complete cycle for the alternating patterns to *take 8 counts* (both the right foot and then left foot lead a 4-count portion of the cycle). Examples shown in Figures 8.26–8.28 are Bench Tap, Floor Tap, and Lunge Back.

- a *step touch*, performed by "touching" the *same* toe or heel on the floor or bench (a 2-count move) or by *alternating* legs (Figure 8.29). Step touch moves often are used during the warm-up to familiarize you with the bench, or as transition moves during the aerobic segment.

For both safety and variety when using the single-lead step, 4-count cycle patterns, lead with the right foot for a *maximum of 1 minute*, then change to a left-foot lead. To accomplish this change in lead foot (for single-cycle 4-count step patterns), perform a *non-weight-bearing, transitional, hold/touch/tap/heel* move as the last step of the cycle, initiating the change with that foot.

Note: Within the figure descriptions, only the moves typeset in boldface are shown in the figures.

SINGLE LEAD STEP

Bench approach: Front (shown), top, end, and diagonal.

FIGURE 8.25 Single Lead Step

	R	L	R	L	
Right Lead:	**Up**	up	down	**down**	(4 counts)

	L	R	L	R	
Left Lead:	Up	up	down	down	(4 counts)

Arms shown: Long-lever punching on up, up; pull, punch, on the down, down.

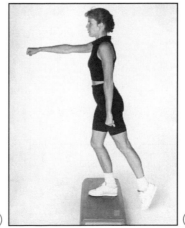

(a)

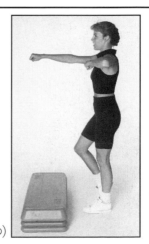

(b)

ALTERNATING LEAD STEP

You can alternate the lead leg with a Bench Tap up (on bench), or a Floor Tap or Lunge Back down (on floor).
Bench approach: Front (shown), top, end, or diagonal.

FIGURE 8.26
Bench Tap

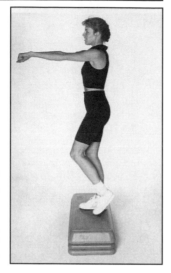

R   L   L   R
Up **bench tap** down down

Alternate: Up (L), bench tap (R), down (R), down (L). (8 counts)

Arms shown: Forward punching.

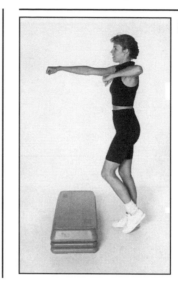

FIGURE 8.27
Floor Tap

R   L   R   L
Up up down **floor tap**

Alternate. (8 counts)

Arms shown: Opposite arm long-lever punching; same arm flexing, elbow kept shoulder high.

Note: The Floor Tap also can be a non-weight-bearing lunge back.

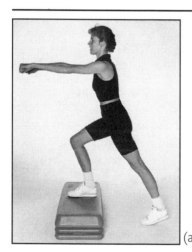
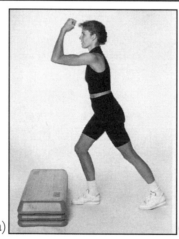

(a)   (b)

FIGURE 8.28   Lunge Back

R   L   R   L
Up up down **down and back**

Alternate. (8 counts)

Arms shown: Arms punching forward and parallel
on up, up; bicep curls keeping elbows still high on the down, down.

STEP TOUCH

You can do the same or alternate the lead leg, touching toe or heel. **Bench approach:** Front (shown), top, end, astride.

FIGURE 8.29   Step Touch

R   R
Bench-tap with toe   down   repeat with left foot. (4 counts)

Arms shown: Elbows shoulder-high, fists together on tap; fists apart on down

OPTIONS:

Try a Bench Tap using the **heel**, instead of the toe.

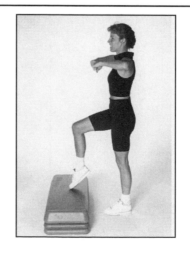
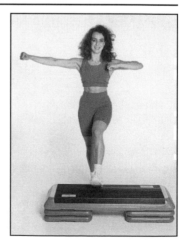

Basic Step Patterns[11]

Basic step patterns may be performed as single lead steps (4-count pattern) or alternating lead steps (8-count pattern).

When performing a single lead basic step pattern, the fourth count of the cycle is weight-bearing.

Alternating lead steps, have two options:

● When the first three steps are weight-bearing, the fourth is non-weight-bearing.

● When the first three steps contain a bypass move, the fourth step is weight-bearing.

Basic step patterns shown include V-step (Figure 8.30), Bypass Variations (Figures 8.31–8.34), and Straddle Up or Down (Figures 8.35–8.36).

FIGURE 8.30   V-Step

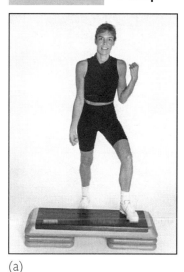
(a)

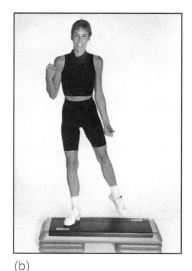
(b)

Bench approach: front

	R	L	R	L
Up-wide	up-wide	**down-center**	down-center

Usually cued: "out" "out" "in" "in".

Arms shown: Same-side single bicep curls.

FIGURE 8.31   Knee Up Bypass[12]

Bench approach : front

	L	R	
Up	**knee lift**	(bypasses the bench and lifts)

	R	L
down (to floor)	down (to floor).

Arms shown: Initiate from arms fully extended out to the sides shoulder high with palms up: Single short-lever curls on the up and knee lift; return one at a time to long-lever, shoulder-high initial position on the down, down.

OPTIONS:

Bench approach side, top, end, diagonal

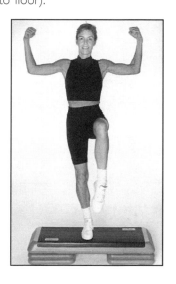

FIGURE 8.32   Kick Forward Bypass

Bench approach: front

L	R	R	L
Up	**kick forward**	down (to floor)	down (to floor).

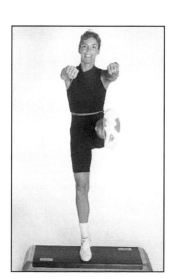

Arms shown: Sweep up arms from sides, together and parallel on up, kick; sweep together and parallel back down to sides on the down, down.

OPTIONS:

Bench approach side, top, end, diagonal

Basic Step Patterns

FIGURE 8.33 **Kick Back Bypass**

Bench approach : front

L	R	
Up	**kick back**	(a "**long lever** raising" motion)
	R	L
	down (to floor)	down (to floor).

Arms shown: Initiate from arms fully extended down at sides: Raise same (one) elbow out wide to shoulder high with fist ending at waist, for the up and kick back; lower to initial position at side with each down, down.

OPTIONS:

Bench approach side, top, end, diagonal

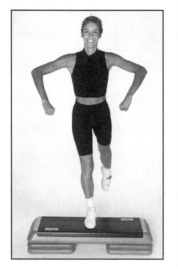

FIGURE 8.34 **Side Leg Lift Bypass**

Bench approach: front

L	R	
Up	**side leg lift**	(a knee pointing forward position),
	R	L
	down (to floor)	down (to floor).

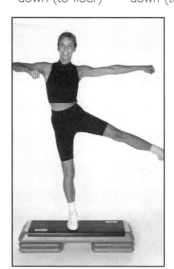

Arms shown: Raise both arms simultaneously to bent-arm lateral raise position for up; same arm (one) extends out to side shoulder high for side leg lift; return extended arm to bent-arm lateral raise on the down; lower both arms simultaneously on the last down.

OPTIONS:

Bench approach side, top, end, diagonal

FIGURE 8.35 **Straddle Up**

Bench approach: astride (shown)

R	L
Up	**knee lift** (bypasses bench and lifts waist high),
L	R
straddle down (to floor)	straddle down (to floor).

Arms shown: Same initial position as last pattern, with opposite arm punching forward on lift.

OPTIONS:

For variety, try the other *bypass moves* (Figures 8.32–8.34), incorporating one or more accompanying arm movements that will keep your balance atop the bench.

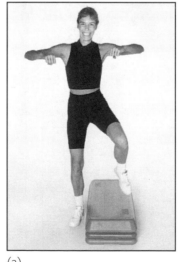

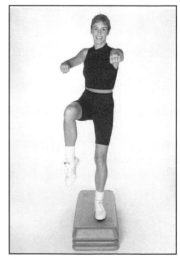

(a)   (b)

Basic Step Patterns

FIGURE 8.36 **Straddle Down**

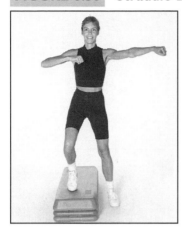 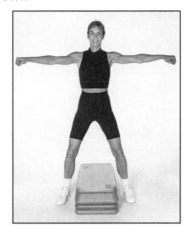

Bench approach: top (shown)

<pre>
                            R
Straddle down (on R side of bench)
                            L
Straddle down (on L side of bench)
            R   L
            Up   Up
</pre>

Arms shown: Shoulder high, short-levers, and fists together at center. Extend same long-lever arm out to side as same leg steps out. Return one arm at a time back in to center on each up, up step.

Variations of Base Steps and Basic Step Patterns

To add interest to base steps and basic step patterns, a number of variations can be implemented. These are categorized here as:

- Traveling (Figures 8.37–8.42)
- Repeaters (Figures 8.43)
- Propulsion (Figure 8.44)
- Adding hand-held weights (Figure 8.45).

TRAVELING PATTERNS

FIGURE 8.37 **Turn Step — Length of the Bench**

Bench approach shown: side

Single lead: 4 counts   Alternating lead: 8 counts

<pre>
     L   R   L   R
    Up   body 1/2 turns left and up   down   tap-down
</pre>

Arms shown: Shoulder high, alternating punch and pull back.

Note: Remember to keep your eyes on the platform. Also, this pattern is shown using natural photography and descriptive words, as it could not be photographed, and therefore described, from a "mirrored" perspective.

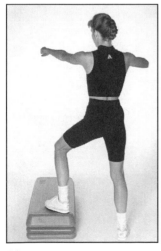 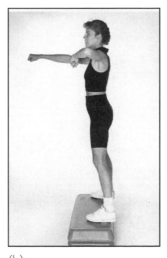 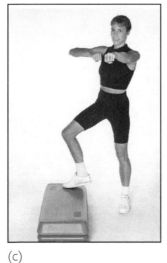 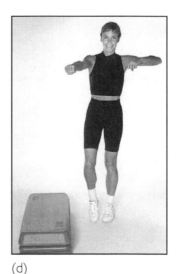

(a)   (b)   (c)   (d)

TRAVELING PATTERNS

FIGURE 8.38   **Over the Top — Width of the Bench**

Bench approach shown: side

Single lead: 4 counts   Alternating lead: 8 counts

L	R	L	R
Up	**up**	**down on the left side of bench/platform**	**touch-down**

Alternate. Cued: "up," "over," "down," "tap"

Arms shown: Elbows pointing skyward and shoulder high, with arms wide open on the first, third, fifth, and seventh steps (a & c); arms low and crossed in front on even-numbered steps (b & d).

OPTIONS:

For variety on the *fourth* step, instead of tapping the floor, touch heel on bench; knee up; or kick front.

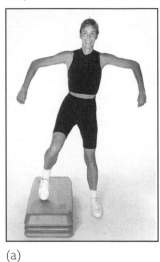
(a)

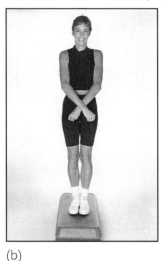
(b)

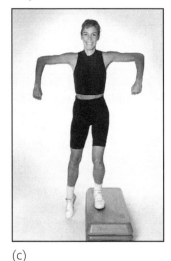
(c)

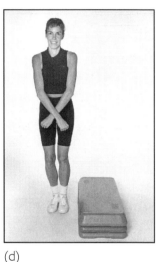
(d)

FIGURE 8.39   **Across the Top — Length of the Bench**

Bench approach shown: end

Single lead: 4 counts   Alternating lead: 8 counts

R	L	R	L
Up	**up**	**down on the right side of bench**	**touch down**

Cued: "up," "across," "down," "tap"

Arms shown: Arms at shoulder level; when legs are apart, arms are straight out to the side (a & c); bend arms into the chest when feet are together (b & d).

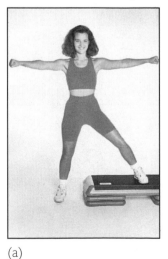
(a)

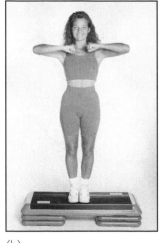
(b)

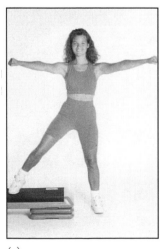
(c)

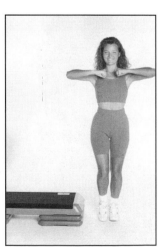
(d)

INTERMEDIATE / ADVANCED VARIATIONS

FIGURE 8.44

Propulsion[14] Steps

In propulsion, both feet push off the ground or bench, exchanging positions during the airborne phase of the pattern. Propulsion steps are commonly used with touch and lunge steps.[15] Propulsion moves also can be used when performing bypass or traveling moves by adding a hop or pushing off the foot on the bench.

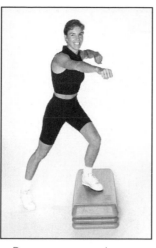

R
Up

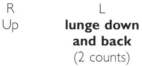

L
lunge down and back
(2 counts)

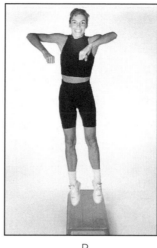

R
Push off (with propulsion into this airborne position)
(1 count)

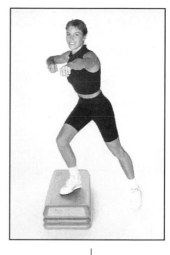

L
Landing on opposite foot up and other foot (R) **lunging down and back** (1 count)

FIGURE 8.45

Step Training Plus Hand-held Weights[16]

Extensive criteria for using hand-held weights were given earlier in this chapter. *Once you are proficient at stepping,* adding 1–4–lb hand-held weights can add intensity and variety to your program. The key to adding hand-held weights to step training is maintaining excellent body positioning throughout and being in absolute control of the weights for all upper-body movements.

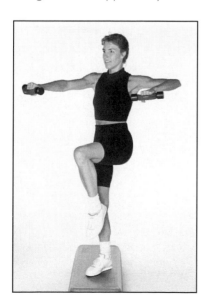

Adding Variety to Base Steps and Basic Step Patterns

To add variety, start with the less intense, low-range motions (elbows kept low, near your waist), and gradually incorporate more intense, middle-range motions (elbows chest-to-shoulder high), and then the highly intense upper-range arm movements (elbows at and above shoulder level).

LOW-RANGE (ELBOW) ARM MOVEMENTS

FIGURE 8.46   Bicep Curls

With elbows **fixed** at the sides, **palms up** (a), flex both elbows, forearms moving toward shoulders (b). For Alternating Bicep Curls, alternate right and left forearms (c).

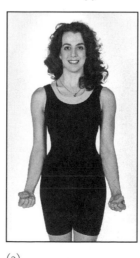

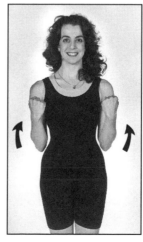

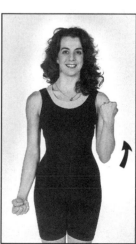

(a)   (b)   (c)

LOW-RANGE (ELBOW) ARM MOVEMENTS

FIGURE 8.47 **Hammer Curls**

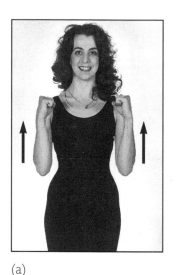 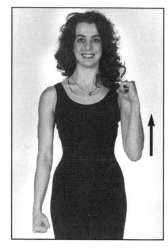

With elbows **fixed** at the sides and **palms facing** each other, flex both elbows, forearms toward the shoulders (a). For Alternating Hammer Curls, alternate right and left forearms (b).

(a)   (b)

FIGURE 8.48

Low Wide 'n Cross

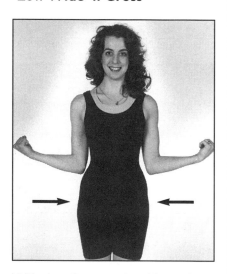

With the elbows at the sides and forearms wide, criss-cross the arms at waist level in front of the body, keeping the palms up. Low punches can be performed by extending both elbows forward away from the body (palms still up), or alternating low punches by extending one forearm at a time.

FIGURE 8.49

Row Low

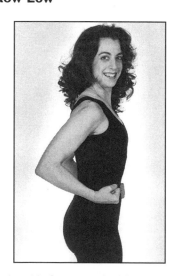

Begin with forearms (only) extended in front of body, waist-level. Pull elbows backward until fists are next to the waist; return to starting position.

FIGURE 8.50

Triceps Kick-Back

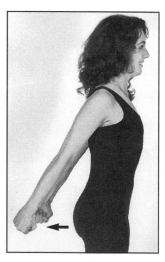

Beginning with the elbows **fixed** behind the shoulders and fists next to sides (Figure 8.49), extend both elbows, forearms moving backward; or alternate right and left arms. Palms can face up/in/down.

MID-RANGE ARM MOVEMENTS

FIGURE 8.51 **Criss-Crossover**

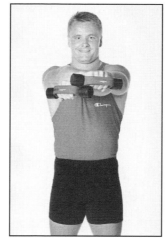
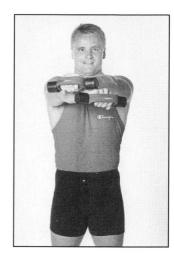

Keeping elbows at chest height, criss-cross the arms over each other, palms facing down (a). Alternate the arm that crosses over the top, for each repetition (b).

(a)   (b)

FIGURE 8.52 **Double and Single Side-Out**

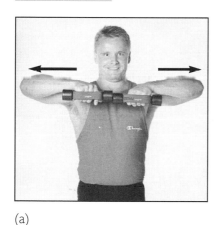
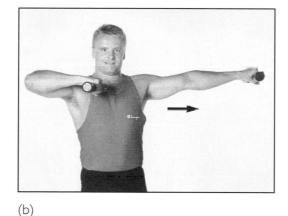

(a)   (b)

Begin with fists under chin at shoulder level, palms down, elbows directly out (a). Extend both arms wide out to the sides, keeping elbows at shoulder height. Pull the fists back into the chin. For single side-outs (b), alternate the right and left arms.

FIGURE 8.53 **Front Shoulder Raises**

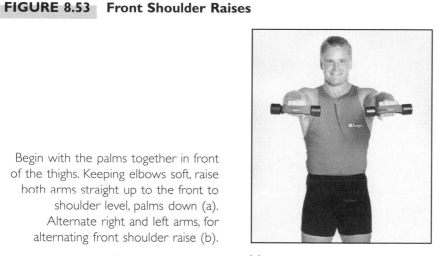
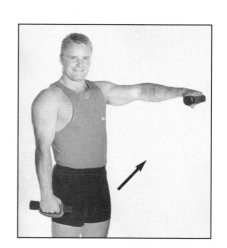

Begin with the palms together in front of the thighs. Keeping elbows soft, raise both arms straight up to the front to shoulder level, palms down (a). Alternate right and left arms, for alternating front shoulder raise (b).

(a)   (b)

FIGURE 8.54 **Upright Row**

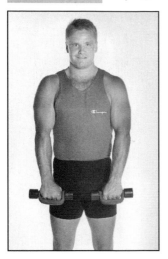

(a)

Begin with the palms in front of the thighs (a). Keeping the fists close to the body and elbows wide, raise the hands up to chin (b).

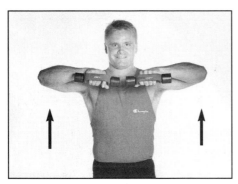

(b)

FIGURE 8.55 **Cross and Lateral Raise**

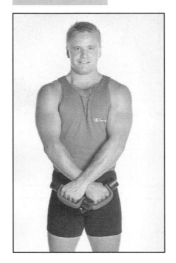

(a)

Begin with arms crossed low in front of abdomen, palms facing body (a). Uncross palms and laterally raise elbows up pointing skyward to shoulder height, keeping arms wide open (b).

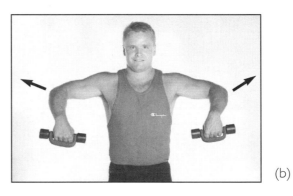

(b)

FIGURE 8.56

Shoulder Punch

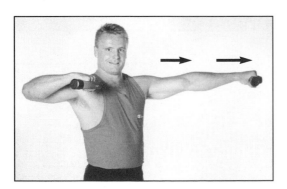

Start with the hands resting lightly on shoulders. Extend one arm forward (a) **or** diagonally across the body, at shoulder height. Pull back and return to shoulder.

FIGURE 8.57

Side Lateral Raise

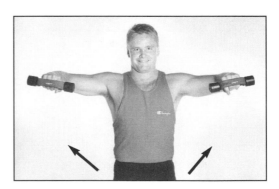

Start with fists together in front of thighs. Lift arms up and out wide, palms facing down, always leading with elbows, keeping them bent slightly.

UPPER-RANGE ARM MOVEMENTS

FIGURE 8.58 **Butterflies**

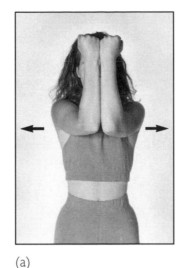

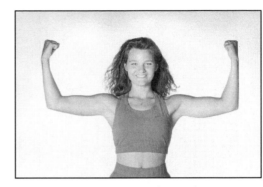

(b)

Begin with fists and forearms together and parallel in front of face, elbows pointing down (a). Keeping elbows shoulder-high, open them wide and out to sides (b).

(a)

FIGURE 8.59 **Slice**

Begin with fists facing and resting on shoulders, elbows low at sides (a). Simultaneously extend one arm upward straight above head while extending other arm downward, alongside of leg (b). Pull both fists back to shoulders, and repeat with other side high/low.

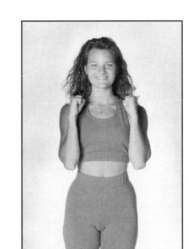

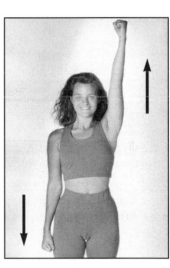

(a)

(b)

FIGURE 8.60 **Side-L**

Begin with fists resting on shoulders (a). Simultaneously extend one arm straight out to side at shoulder height while extending the other arm upward above the head (b). Pull both fists back to shoulders and repeat, other direction.

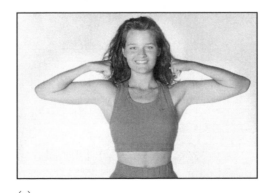

(a)

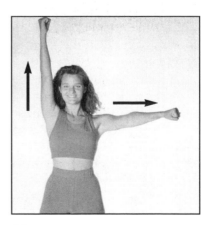

(b)

FIGURE 8.61
Front-L

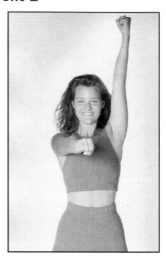

Start with fists resting on shoulders (see Figure 8.60 a). Simultaneously extend one arm straight out in front of you, shoulder height, while extending other arm upward above head. Pull both fists back to shoulders and repeat, other direction.

FIGURE 8.62
Overhead Press

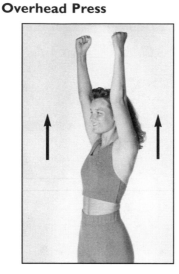

Start with fists resting on shoulders (see Figure 8.60 a). With palms facing, extend arms upward over head, keeping elbows close to ears. For alternating overhead press, alternate right and left arms.

FIGURE 8.63
Triceps Extension

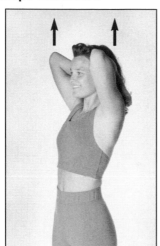

Begin with elbows fixed high, near ears and fists on shoulders. With palms facing, extend arms high and parallel overhead (see Figure 8.62).

Applying The Techniques

Create an 8- or 16-count step pattern that utilizes all three sides of the bench, beginning from the end of the bench. When you get creative, do not ever have your back facing the bench while stepping up. Use only three sides of the bench for any one pattern, for safety reasons.

Steps from the end use multiple bench-approaches and multiple basic step patterns. Try the sample pattern diagrammed in Figure 8.64.

The figure illustrates an empty bench with sequential placement location of each foot. Beginning from the bench's end and with your weight on your right foot on the floor, step up on bench to the #1 location with your left foot. Continue on with the pattern, placing your next foot atop, on the side, or at the end, and on the floor, wherever the sequential number indicates for foot placement.

When alternating the pattern, final step 16 is a step (taking weight onto left foot). The next move is up (right). And, when creating a totally new pattern, final step 16 is a non-weight-bearing move (like a "tap"), with the next weight-bearing step on that same ("tap") foot, either in place on the floor, or up, on the bench.

FIGURE 8.64   From the End

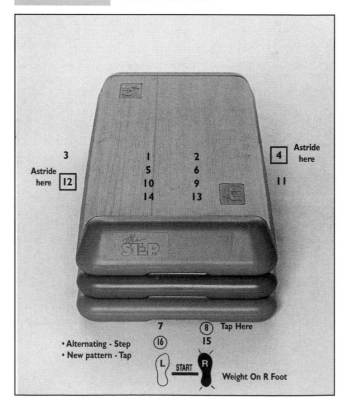

CREATING YOUR OWN STEP TRAINING PATTERN VARIATIONS

Following all of the guidelines you've been given, you will be able to create your own patterns. Start with a bench approach from the end, front, side, or top, and proceed, incorporating multiple basic step patterns and multiple bench approaches. Use the form, Figure 8.65, to:

● Indicate the location of the weight-bearing foot (WBF) to start the pattern, freeing the other foot to then be step #1. The bench and floor have been divided into six sections for your convenience in placing the number locations.

● Begin the pattern by locating a "1" up on the bench (or down on the floor), followed by the location of the next step, identified as "2."

● Continue locating steps 3–8, then 9–16, identifying any step that has a key directive (e.g., ⑧ is a tap non-weight-bearing move; ⑫ is an astride position).

● Identify any bypass step movement with a double circle around the non-weight-bearing foot location and labeling the type of bypass move (e.g., ⑤ forward kick).

● List arm gestures to accompany each step movement, plus any additional choreographed pointers (sounds, etc.) at the right. Enjoy being creative!

Possible steps and variations available to you are summarized in Figure 8.66. As you begin to develop an individualized program, you can incorporate your favorite step training moves in the combinations you choose.

FIGURE 8.65 **Creating Your Own Patterns**

Steps:

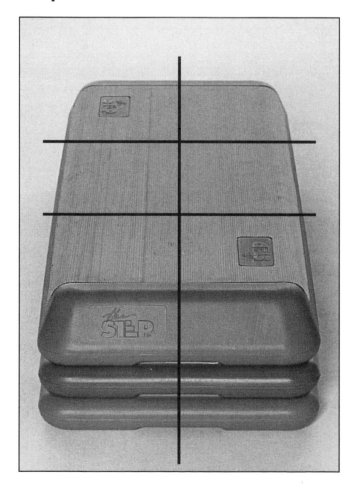

Arm Gestures to Step #:

1. _____
2. _____
3. _____
4. _____
5. _____
6. _____
7. _____
8. _____
9. _____
10. _____
11. _____
12. _____
13. _____
14. _____
15. _____
16. _____

FIGURE 8.65 Continued

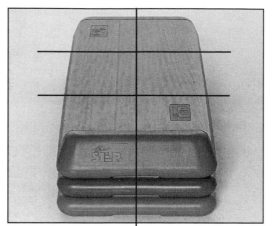

1._____	9._____
2._____	10._____
3._____	11._____
4._____	12._____
5._____	13._____
6._____	14._____
7._____	15._____
8._____	16._____

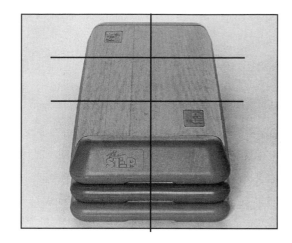

1._____	9._____
2._____	10._____
3._____	11._____
4._____	12._____
5._____	13._____
6._____	14._____
7._____	15._____
8._____	16._____

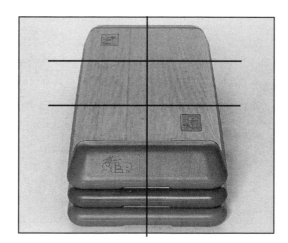

1._____	9._____
2._____	10._____
3._____	11._____
4._____	12._____
5._____	13._____
6._____	14._____
7._____	15._____
8._____	16._____

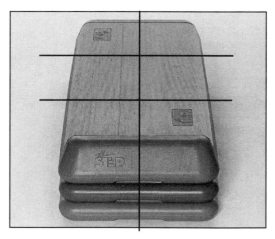

1._____	9._____
2._____	10._____
3._____	11._____
4._____	12._____
5._____	13._____
6._____	14._____
7._____	15._____
8._____	16._____

FIGURE 8.66 **Summary of Step Training Techniques**[17]

1. DIRECTION your body faces the bench
   - Front
   - End
   - Side
   - Top
   - Astride/Straddle
   - Diagonal

2. Then as

BASE STEPS
- Single lead step
- Alternating lead step
  - Bench tap
  - Floor tap
  - Lunge back
- Step touch
  - With toe
  - With heel

BASIC STEP PATTERNS
- V-Step
- Bypass variations
  - Knee-up bypass
  - Kick-forward bypass
  - Kick-backward bypass
  - Side-leg lift bypass
- Straddle up
  - With all bypasses mentioned above
- Straddle down

Then can be:

VARIATIONS OF BASE STEPS AND BASIC STEP PATTERNS
- Traveling Patterns
  - Turn step – length of bench
  - Over the top – width of bench, 4th step a:
    - Tap on floor
    - Touch heel on bench
    - Knee up
    - Kick front
  - Across the top – length of bench
    - With same options as above
  - Diagonal to diagonal
    - Variety on 2nd and 6th steps: any bypass move
  - Inside end to outside end
  - Around the corner
- Repeaters
  - With taps
  - With any bypass move
- Propulsion
  - With lunge steps
  - With bypasses – add a hop
  - With traveling steps – add a hop
- Adding hand-held weights

Also
- Aerobics and Step Training
- Step and Strength Training

VARIATIONS OF BASIC ARM MOVEMENTS
- Low-/mid-/upper-range
  - Arm movements
    – Low (double/alternating arms)
  - Bicep curls
  - Hammer curls
  - Low wide 'n cross
  - Row low
  - Triceps kick-back
    – Mid-(double/alternating arms)
  - Criss-crossover
  - Side-out
  - Front shoulder raises
  - Shoulder punch
  - Diagonal shoulder punch
  - Side lateral raise
  - Upright row
  - Cross and lateral raise
    – Upper –
  - Butterflies (double/alternating arms)
  - Slice
  - Side-L
  - Front-L
  - Overhead press (double/alternating arms)
  - Triceps extension (double/alternating arms)

© Morton Publishing Company, Karen S. Mazzeo

Goal Setting Challenge

Set a short-term goal to develop at least one new 16-count pattern you enjoy each week. Then set a course-goal to use your created new patterns together in a sequence that lasts as long as your favorite step training song.

Developing Goal Scripts for Chapter 8

DIRECTIONS: Write complete sentences for each segment below. Combine your responses to all four segments. This goal script is designed around your needs and choices. Read it (or make an audiotape and play it) twice daily, morning and evening, until you master it.

1 State one goal in positive, *present-tense* language. Ask yourself, "What will I experience — see, hear, taste, smell, feel — in regard to the results? Keep in mind that all powerful goals use the SMART formula: specific, measurable, achievable, realistic, timely.

_____

_____

2 State your *pleasure-value reasons*. Ask yourself, "Why am I totally committed to achieving this goal? What am I choosing to feel?"

_____

_____

3 State your *pain-avoidance value reasons*. Ask yourself, "What painful values do I choose to avoid feeling?"

_____

_____

4 State *immediate action(s)* you can take in the next 24 hours. Use positive, present-tense verbs such as *choose* and verbs ending with "ing."

_____

_____

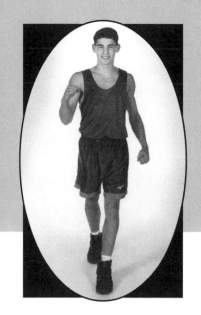

Aerobic Exercise: Fitness Walking and Jumping Rope (Option 3)

Fitness walking is probably the easiest of all aerobic options because it can be done anywhere with no need for equipment or another's direction. Because it takes three times as long to get the same aerobic benefits from walking as from running,[1] *time* is a key factor when planning variety. Exercise action taking *14 minutes or longer per mile is classified as walking*, taking 9–12 minutes per mile is labeled *jogging*, and taking under 9 minutes per mile is *running*.[2]

SHOES AND APPAREL

Supportive walking or running shoes are important to cushion and absorb the impact that walking provides (see Table 3.1 in Chapter 3). Because one foot is always on the ground, fitness walking is classified as a low-impact activity.

Clothing worn is loose and comfortable, pants not too baggy or too long to interfere with motion and ground contact. When temperatures are 40° F. or below, your air passages are always covered with appropriate clothing.

PRINCIPLES AND TECHNIQUES

The initial body position is the same as it is for standing (see Figure 4.4 in Chapter 4), except that as the legs swing forward, a new base of support is established with each swing and the center of gravity moves forward, over the base. The body weight is balanced, *slightly forward*. The breathing pattern is easy and continuous while you move quickly.

MECHANICS

The sequence of movements is as follows.

1. Swing the legs forward with the hip/thigh leading until the heel strikes the ground (with a minimum of lateral or vertical movement).

2. As the heel touches down (Figure 9.1), push off the back leg from the ball of the foot and the big toe area (Figure 9.2), transferring the weight to the first foot.

3. Swing the back leg easily under the body as the base of support is formed. Keep the body in a balanced position so a change of direction can occur.

The balanced position is supported by strong leg muscles, which allow the weight shift to the heel of the first foot to be smooth and controlled. Many people, however, use the back muscles instead of the leg muscles to lead and support the body. The center of gravity (center of your weight) is then ahead of the base of support, which puts the trunk in an unsupported position

FIGURE 9.1

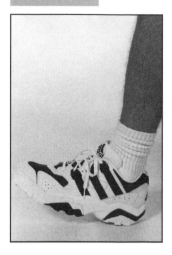

Leading with heel.

FIGURE 9.2

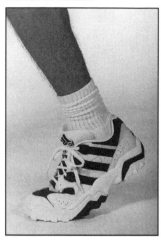

Pushing off with ball of foot.

and leads to early fatigue and back pain. Think *relaxed lower back*.

4. Position and make ground contact with feet as follows:

   a. Touch center of the heel first.

   b. With a rolling action forward, shift your weight through the center and outer half of the foot (Figure 9.3).

   c. Push off from the ball of the foot and the big toe.

   d. Point the feet straight ahead and place them just to the left and right of an imaginary center line.

5. Keeping the shoulders level and parallel, swing

FIGURE 9.3

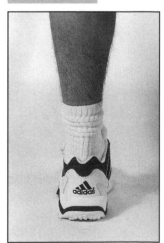

Shifting weight through outer half of foot.

the arms freely and naturally and in opposition to the forward leg, in one of these two positions:

a. Hold arms in a *long-lever*, relaxed-elbow position (Figure 9.4), with a forward and backward controlled swinging motion that also involves upper torso conditioning.

b. Hold arms in a *short-lever* position, elbows flexed and held near sides (Figure 9.5). Hold hands in a relaxed first with either arm position.

FITNESS WALKING PROGRAM

Table 9.1 presents a Level I, 10-Week Walking Program.[3] It is easy to follow and can be enjoyed anywhere. Note that proper warm-up and cool-down ("warm down") are required for a safe program.

FIGURE 9.4

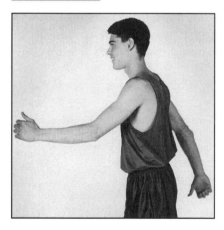

Long-lever position.

FIGURE 9.5

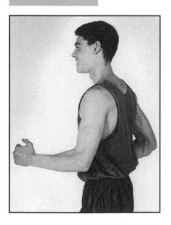

Short-lever elbow position.

TABLE 9.1   LEVEL 1: WALKING ONLY*

Week	Session	Warm Up	Exercise	Warm Down	Goal (Distance)
1	1	yes	15-20'	yes	0.5 to 0.8 mi.
	2	yes	15-20'	yes	0.9 to 1.0 mi.
	3	yes	20'	yes	0.9 to 1.0 mi.
2	4	yes	20'	yes	0.9 to 1.0 mi.
	5	yes	24'	yes	1.1 to 1.2 mi.
	6	yes	24'	yes	1.1 to 1.2 mi.
3	7	yes	28'	yes	1.3 to 1.4 mi.
	8	yes	28'	yes	1.3 to 1.4 mi.
	9	yes	32'	yes	1.4 to 1.6 mi.
4	10	yes	32'	yes	1.4 to 1.6 mi.
	11	yes	36'	yes	1.7 to 1.8 mi.
	12	yes	36'	yes	1.7 to 1.8 mi.
5	13	yes	40'	yes	1.9 to 2.0 mi.
	14	yes	40'	yes	1.9 to 2.0 mi.
	15	yes	44'	yes	2.1 to 2.2 mi.
6	16	yes	48'	yes	2.3 to 2.4 mi.
	17	yes	48'	yes	2.3 to 2.4 mi.
	18	yes	48'	yes	2.3 to 2.4 mi.
7	19	yes	52'	yes	2.5 to 2.6 mi.
	20	yes	52'	yes	2.5 to 2.6 mi.
	21	yes	56'	yes	2.7 to 2.8 mi.
8	22	yes	56'	yes	2.7 to 2.8 mi.
	23	yes	60'	yes	2.9 to 3.0 mi.
	24	yes	60'	yes	2.9 to 3.0 mi.
9	25	yes	58'	yes	3.0 mi.
	26	yes	58'	yes	3.0 mi.
	27	yes	56'	yes	3.0 mi.
10	28	yes	56'	yes	3.0 mi.
	29	yes	54'	yes	3.0 mi.
	30	yes	54'	yes	3.0 mi.

*Program written by Dr. Richard Bowers, ACSM certified Program Director

LIFETIME WALKING PROGRAM

If you have access to a recreational facility that has a *pace trail*, you can add another element to your fitness program: challenging yourself to improve your cardiovascular fitness continually by using the permanently visible measurement device built into the trail that quantifies time and distance covered.

This trail has outdoor safety lighting poles at premeasured distances. Each is equipped with a bank of mechanized, color-coded, flashing lights. These colored lights have been synchronized to flash at regular timed intervals, reflecting specific minutes-per-mile covered (see Figure 9.6). Arriving at a pole as the specific colored light you've chosen to follow is flashing reflects that you are covering a predetermined distance in a predetermined time. It is a helpful means to stay focused on fitness results and continued improvement.

RESEARCH DATA TO ASSIST WITH SETTING GOALS

Research conducted at the Cooper Institute in Dallas[4] demonstrated that walking at a moderate pace of 3 miles per hour (a 20-minute mile) increased cardiovascular fitness and reduced the risk of heart disease by increasing the HDL- ("good") cholesterol (see

FIGURE 9.6   **Pace Trail to Help Keep Focus on Goals**

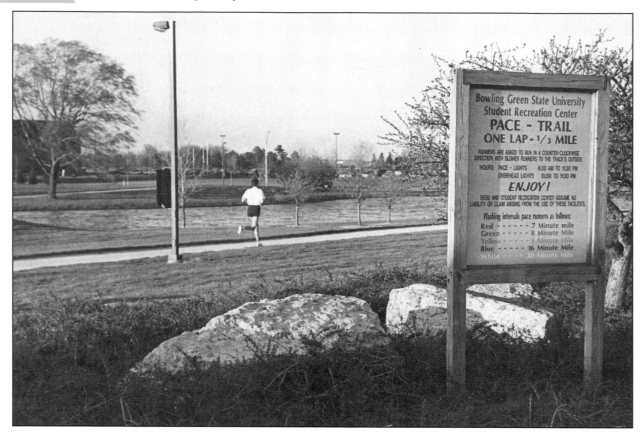

Chapter 14). Walking a 12-minute mile resulted in a greater improvement in fitness levels than for the 20-minute-per-mile group but similar increases in HDL-cholesterol. This demonstrated that you don't have to do vigorous activity to get a health benefit.

Also, *you don't have to do all your activity in one session.* Studies show that you can get almost the same benefit from three 10-minute exercise bouts as one 30-minute exercise bout of equal intensity. Most people can find time to take a brisk walk for 2, 5, or 10 minutes several times during the day. Minimum amounts of exercise to achieve results are given in Table 9.2.

> *Younger people probably need to do a bit more, and older people could do a bit less than the typical program.*

TABLE 9.2   **Minimum Exercise Needed**

	Women	Men
For "moderate" exercise	Walk 2 miles in less than 30 minutes (a 15 minute mile) at least three days per week, or walk 2 miles in 30 to 40 minutes (a 15–20 minute mile) five to six times per week.	Walk 2 miles in less than 27 minutes (a 13½ minute mile) at least three days per week, or walk 2 miles in 30 to 40 minutes (a 15–20 minute mile) six to seven times per week.
For "high fitness"	Walk 2 miles in less than 30 minutes five or six days per week.	Walk 2½ miles in less than 37½ minutes six to seven days per week.

JUMPING ROPE

Jumping rope is a strenuous activity that uses approximately three times more energy than leisure walking. This high-impact activity is not suited for everyone. Inactive individuals and those with joint and back problems should not participate in this form of aerobic exercise. Others with exercise experience should have no problem.

A giving surface upon which to jump is preferable. The rope should reach your armpits, when held down tightly under your feet, with a few extra inches, or a handle, with which to hold the rope comfortably (Figure 9.7). If no handles are present, tape the ends or tie knots at the ends to prevent fraying. Among the variety of jump ropes on the market are beaded, licorice, leather, and cotton ropes. Beaded ropes and leather ropes are the best choice. Licorice (plastic) ropes get tangled more frequently, and cotton ropes are rather difficult to use because they are so lightweight.

The following procedure is recommended for jumping rope:

1. When you warm up, be sure to static-stretch all the muscles of the leg, with special attention to the calf, heel cord, and shin areas.

2. Begin the aerobic segment with 6 minutes, progressing up to a 20-minute workout. Jump low with "soft" knees for efficiency, and only high enough to clear the rope (less than 1").

3. Restrict continuous jumping to 1-minute intervals at 120–140 revolutions per minute, a moderate pace. Alternate 1-minute segments with non-jumping low-impact aerobics such as marching or power walking. Music should range from 120–140 beats per minute also, to assist in timing and rhythm.

4. Use rate of perceived exertion to monitor your intensity because it will allow you a minute-to-minute monitoring of how you feel.

5. Provide a 5–10 minute cool-down, including nonjumping, low-impact moves, and flexibility and relaxation for 5 minutes, static stretching again for the leg muscles used.[5]

OPTIONS:

- One foot and then the other (Figure 9.8). Don't do more than four repetitions on the same foot. Alternate immediately to the other foot for the same number of steps.
- Two feet at a time (Figure 9.9).
- Jumping with arm/rope crossed, followed by a one-footed or two-footed jump.
- Hopscotch jump: using a two-foot jump astride, one-foot jump, two-foot jump astride, alternate one-foot jump.

FIGURE 9.7

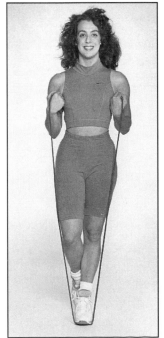

Correct length of rope.

FIGURE 9.8

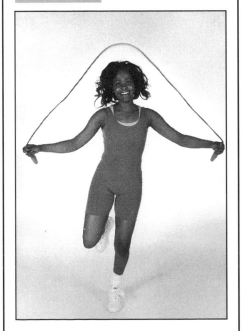

One-footed rope jumping.

FIGURE 9.9

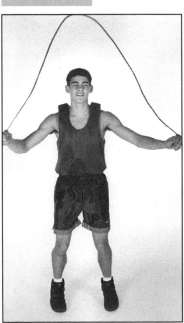

Two-footed rope jumping.

Goal Setting Challenge

Set a short-term goal and a long-range goal that incorporate variety in a fitness walking program to help with your fitness commitment for a lifetime.

If you are a candidate for high-impact aerobic exercise, add variety to your program by setting a goal to incorporate at least one rope jumping segment to your workouts.

Developing Goal Scripts for Chapter 9

DIRECTIONS: Write complete sentences for each segment below. Combine your responses to all four segments. This goal script is designed around your needs and choices. Read it (or make an audiotape and play it) twice daily, morning and evening, until you master it.

❶ State one goal in positive, *present-tense* language. Ask yourself, "What will I experience — see, hear, taste, smell, feel — in regard to the results? Keep in mind that all powerful goals use the SMART formula: specific, measurable, achievable, realistic, timely.

_____

_____

❷ State your *pleasure-value reasons*. Ask yourself, "Why am I totally committed to achieving this goal? What am I choosing to feel?"

_____

_____

❸ State your *pain-avoidance value reasons*. Ask yourself, "What painful values do I choose to avoid feeling?"

_____

_____

❹ State *immediate action(s)* you can take in the next 24 hours. Use positive, present-tense verbs such as *choose* and verbs ending with "ing."

_____

_____

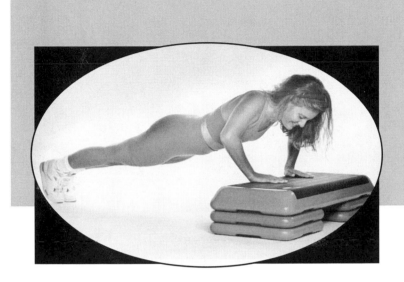

Strength Training

Although all the muscles of the body are strengthened during vigorous aerobic exercise, the optional strength program included within a fitness session focuses on *strength development of isolated muscle groups*. It comes at the *end* of the aerobic exercise segment but before the final cool-down, flexibility training, and relaxation segment.

The reasoning for this is simple. With an increase in the resistance (weight) that must be applied to any movement for significant change to occur, the workload placed on the heart, lungs, and vascular system also increases. An individual is placed more readily in a breathless "oxygen-debt" state. During the aerobic phase your goal is *not* to be in a breathless state. You want to be working continually in a breathe-easy state, steadily pacing your intensity.

The isolation exercises/strength training segment focuses on specific muscle groups in a steady, controlled manner, *concentrating on areas not worked adequately during the aerobic segment*. In contrast to aerobics and step training, which are lower-body intensive, this segment works primarily the muscles in the upper body and the abdominals.

Strength-training exercises are done to more quickly define, tone, shape, and make more dense (thicken) the muscle fibers. They also allow longer periods of work during the exercise program and later in daily work tasks. To incorporate variety into the strength training segment, different forms of resistance, such as hand-held weights, resistance bands, and tubing, can be used. Principles, guidelines, and suggested exercises for safe, effective strength training follow.

PRINCIPLES OF STRENGTH TRAINING

Because the focus is now on resistance work, which is best done when the body is thoroughly warm, the timeframe becomes optional and is according to your priorities in your workout session. If possible, plan approximately 10–20 minutes for strength training during your fitness class, following these principles:

- Precede and follow muscle strengthening exercises by stretching exercises specific for the muscles that are made to work against resistance. Any muscle group strengthened by exercise also should be stretched regularly to prevent abnormal contraction of resting length.[1]

- Of key importance, stabilize your joints and your spine before beginning each exercise.

- Perform each movement using a smooth, continuous, full range-of-motion action for the joint/muscle group involved, and keep the timing of the movement (usually slow) totally under your control. Ballistic (rapid or jerky) movements increase the risk of injury.

- Take approximately 2 seconds to perform the overcoming-resistance (concentric) phase, and 2–4 seconds (i.e., at least the same time, or up to twice as long) during the release or lowering (eccentric) phase to return to the starting position of each exercise.[2]

- Exhale during the lifting, overcoming-resistance-action move; inhale during the release or lowering and return. (Exception: During overhead pressing movements, inhale as you lift.)[3]

- Engage in visualization and self-talk here (see Chapters 2 and 12). Plan your concentrated thoughts to accompany your lifting/exhale and lowering/ inhale movements.

- Follow the progressive resistance format. Begin with one to three sets of 8–12 repetitions for most exercises. (Exception: For abdominal work, begin your program by performing two sets of 15–30 repetitions per set). Select 8–10 exercises that condition the major muscle groups of your body for at least two of your fitness class sessions per week, if you have no other separate strength training program.

- When you become jerky, are not smooth, continuous, and rhythmical in the move, and are not using the full range-of-motion possible around your joints, stop. You've completed your lower limit for that set. This lower limit becomes your baseline to which you attempt to add more repetitions as soon as possible.

- Add resistance in increasingly greater increments (1–4 pounds if using hand weights, or thicker rubber if using bands/tubing). In the fitness class setting, don't go over the 4-pound limit for hand-held weights if this is your choice of resistance equipment.

- Do strength training of isolated muscle groups *every-other-day*. Your muscles need a day to recover, so don't incorporate a program to strength train with resistance (weights/bands/ tubing) daily. As an alternative to this program, perform strength training exercises with resistance (weights/bands/tubing) for the upper half of your body one day and for the lower half of your body the next day. Thus, you are alternating the days that the muscles are strength training.

- Allow brief rest periods between bouts of vigorous exercises. The timeframe for *rest* is defined as *regaining a normal breathing pattern*.

- To incorporate variety into your program, try using all of the forms of resistance illustrated in this chapter:

  1. Your own body (or parts) lifted and lowered against gravity as the weight resistance used, as in push-ups (chapter opening photo) or curl-ups. To progressively increase the resistance involved in lifting your body's weight against gravity, use a strategically placed free-weight (on the sternum for a curl-up, Figure 10.21a, or between the shoulder blades for a push-up, and so on).

  2. Hand-held weights (not wrist-weights) in controlled movement or placed on the body in the key locations to add weight resistance to the body part being lifted and lowered.

  3. Rubber resistance *bands*, 9", 12", or 16" long, in widths of ¼"–1½ inches. The length and width are selected according to whether the exercise works the upper or lower body, and your current strength fitness level in the muscle group being trained.

  4. Rubber resistance *tubing*, approximately 3'–4½ feet long, so you can adjust it according to your height in a range of light to heavy thickness that you select according to your current strength level.

  5. All the above combined, using a step bench in a level position, or in the gravity-assisted incline or decline positions.*

From the exercises presented in this chapter, you will begin to realize that the possibilities for *variety* in your strength training segment are fun, exciting, inexpensive, and unlimited.

Options 3, 4, and 5 are all illustrated in Figure 10.1. Following are the principles for using these unique pieces of equipment.

Using Resistance Bands and Tubing

General principles for using either resistance bands or tubing include the following:

- Select bands and tubing based on your fitness level.

---

*The bench is not designed for using free-weights of more than 10 pounds.[4] For comfort and safety, place a towel on the bench platform when lying on it.

FIGURE 10.1

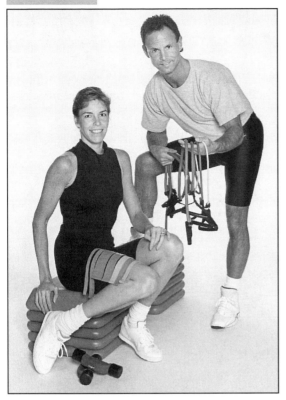

Various equipment to use for resistance.

- Before each use, inspect the bands and tubing for nicks and tears that may arise from continued use.
- Never, under any circumstances, tie pieces of band and tubing together.
- Always exhibit proper body alignment and posture while exercising, as illustrated in the figures in this chapter.
- Keep your face turned slightly away from the direction of movement, for safety.
- While performing single-limb, upper body movements, always anchor the band between one hand and the thigh, hip, side, or shoulder, depending on the movement.
- Always anchor the tubing under the ball of one foot or both feet, depending on your level of fitness and the desired amount of tension.
- Always control the bands and tubing, especially during the return phase of the movement. Do not let them control you.
- Perform 8–10 repetitions of each exercise. When using one arm or one leg, switch sides so the same muscle group is worked an equal

number of repetitions on the opposite side of the body. Be sure to work all muscular groups with equal intensity and repetitions at each session, to avoid muscular imbalance.[5]

Specifics of Bands

Bands (Figures 10.2 and 10.3) are available in a variety of sizes to change the intensity of your workout.[6] Suggested sizes are:

- **Beginner**
  3/8" upper body (pink)
  3/8" (pink) or 5/8" (light blue) lower body
- **Intermediate**
  5/8" upper body (light blue)
  5/8" lower body
- **Advanced**
  3/4" upper body (dark blue)
  3/4" lower body

FIGURE 10.2

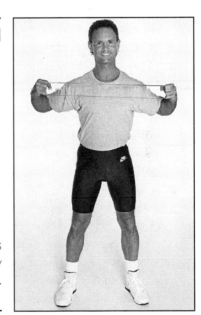

Using resistance bands for upper body (deltoid press-away).

FIGURE 10.3

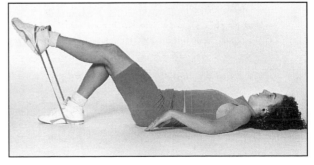

Using resistance bands for lower body (leg extension for quadriceps).

Specifics of Tubing

Tubing also is available in a variety of sizes to change the intensity of your workout.[7] Suggested sizes are:

- **Beginner**
  Very light (yellow) and light tubing (green)
- **Intermediate**
  Light (green) and medium tubing (red)
- **Advanced**
  Heavy tubing (blue)

All of the tubing exercises described in this chapter are designed for the beginner and intermediate exerciser. This means that one foot always will be placed on the center of the tubing to create resistance. You can use the other foot to anchor the tubing if you like. Participants who want to create more resistance stand on the tubing with both feet. The wider you spread your feet, the more resistance you will create (Figures 10.4-10.6).[8]

GUIDELINES FOR STRENGTH TRAINING

Because strength and endurance are considered together as a vital component of total physical well-being, most fitness classes today include a 10–20 minute segment on strength training the skeletal muscles. Guidelines from the American College of Sports Medicine state:

> Strength training of a moderate intensity, sufficient to develop and maintain fat-free weight, should be an integral part of an adult fitness program. One set of eight to twelve repetitions, of eight to ten exercises that condition the major muscle groups, at least two days per week, is the recommended minimum.[9]

Thus, the prescription for more fully developing your lean (fat-free) weight is:

Set	Reps	Varieties of Exercises	Minimum Days/Week
1	8–12	8–10 targeting major muscle groups	2 (with max.: 4/week, or every other day)

You'll be focusing on the following isolated muscle groups of the upper, mid, and lower body.

- Upper body: chest, upper back, shoulders, and arms.
- Mid-section: abdominals, lower back.
- Lower body: hips and buttocks, thighs, and lower legs.

FIGURE 10.4

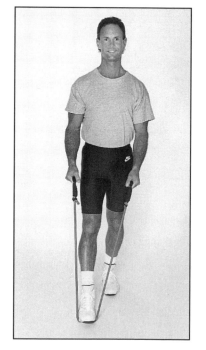

Beginner: one foot on tubing.

FIGURE 10.5

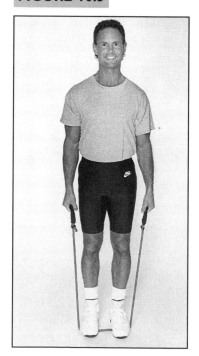

Intermediate: both feet on tubing.

FIGURE 10.6

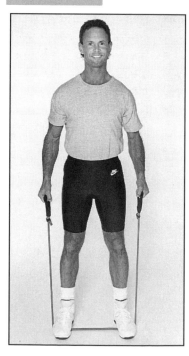

Advanced: feet spread on tubing.

The exercises illustrated and described here have been categorized according to the location of the muscle group(s) benefited (upper body/mid-section/lower body) using a variety of equipment. Breathe evenly on all strength-training exercises. Do not hold your breath. Your working muscles need oxygen constantly. Figure 10.7 illustrates the major muscle groups to be strength-trained,[10] and Table 10.1 identifies, in the order of their presentation, the exercises that will accomplish the training.

FIGURE 10.7 Major Muscles to be Strength-Trained

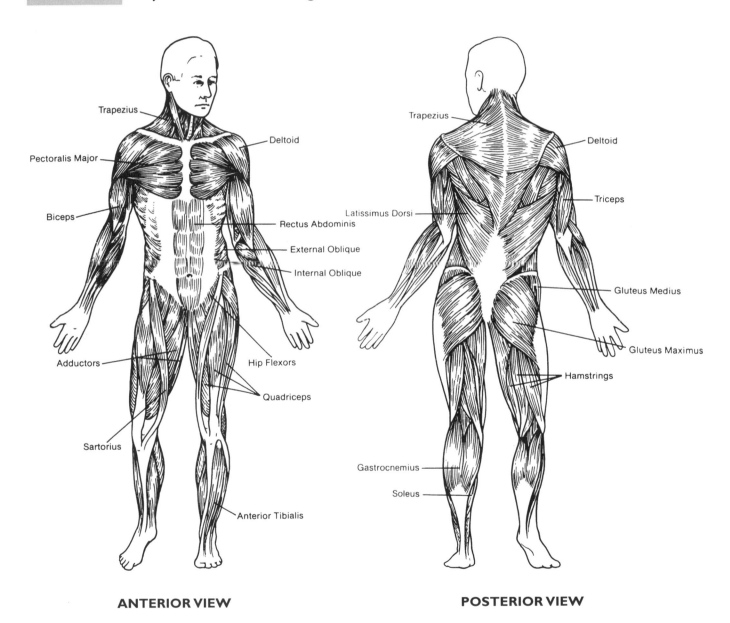

ANTERIOR VIEW   **POSTERIOR VIEW**

TABLE 10.1   Strength Training Exercises Using Various Forms of Resistance[11, 12, 13]

UPPER BODY
Chest/Upper Back/Shoulders/Arms

- Bent-Arm Chest Cross-Over (bench and tubing) (Figure 10.8)
- Push-Up Variations (Figure 10.9)
- Flyes–Variations (weights/tubing) (Figure 10.10)
- Chest (Pec) Cross-Over (tubing) (Figure 10.11)
- Seated Lat Row (tubing) (Figure 10.12)
- Lat Pull-Down (tubing) (Figure 10.13)
- Deltoid Lateral Raise (tubing/weights) (Figure 10.14)
  - With/without Squats (bench/tubing)
- Upright Row (bench and tubing) (Figure 10.15)
- Bicep Curls (tubing/double tubing/weights/band) (Figure 10.16)
  - With Squat (bench and tubing)
- Triceps Kick (Press) Back (band/tubing) (Figure 10.17)
- Triceps Extension (tubing) (Figure 10.18)
- Overhead Press (tubing/bench and tubing) (Figure 10.19)

MID-SECTION
Abdominals/Low Back

- Back Extension (incline bench) (Figure 10.20)
- Gravity-Assisted Curl-Up (weights/incline bench) (Figure 10.21)
  - Reverse Curl-Up (decline bench)
  - Curl-Up Variation

LOWER BODY
Hips and Buttocks/Thighs/Lower Legs

- Squats (bench/weights) (Figure 10.22)
- Buttocks/Heel Lift (band) (Figure 10.23)
- Side Leg Raise (band) (Figure 10.24)
- Inner Thigh Lift (band) (Figure 10.25)
- Leg Curl (band) (Figure 10.26)
- Heel Raise with Squat (bench and tubing) (Figure 10.27)
- Seated Lower Leg Flexor and Extensor (tubing) (Figures 3.6–3.7)

FIGURE 10.8   Bent-Arm Chest Cross-Over

(Pectorals)

OPTION 1:   Bench and Tubing

Position: Sit center, move buttocks to lower third of bench, lie with head resting at top. Grab tube under platform at top block where it is grooved. Feet flat on floor, knees in open position.

OPTION 2:   Tubing and Aerobics

Position: Standing with bent knees, one heel forward and one foot back. Tube across the back, under armpits, and open wide, with bent arms. Roll the tube up around your hands for correct tube length (c).

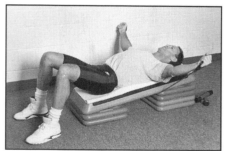

(a)

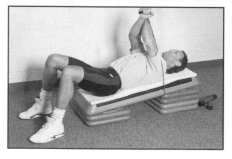

(b)

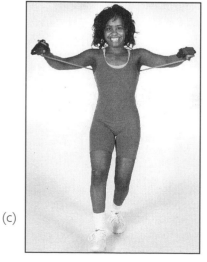

(c)

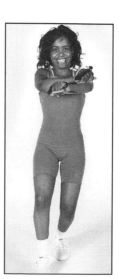

(d)

Action: Cross-punch arm position over chest, from (b) or (d).

FIGURE 10.9 Push-Ups
(Pectorals)

OPTION 1: Static Push-Up

Position: Men and women alike perform a static push-up for as long as possible. This is done by lowering the body until the arms are flexed to 90° or less (2" or 3" above the floor) (a). Keep the entire body straight and off the floor, with the exception of hands and feet.

Action: Use a timer and record the *number of seconds the position is held in this position.* (Exercise is over when abdomen drops or arms straighten.)

OPTION 2: Push-Up

Position: Perform as many continuous push-ups as possible. Keeping the body straight, the chest must touch the floor each time, and arms must be fully extended at the end of each repetition (b).

Action: One rep is counted each time you complete cycle and return up to full arm extension. Record the *number of continuous reps* (in good form, until muscle exhaustion) as one set.

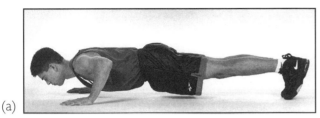

(a)

Arms flexed to 90° or less.

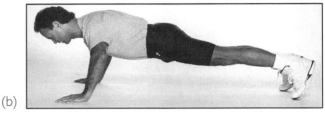

(b)

Arms fully extended at end of rep.

OPTION 3: Bench Push-Up See chapter opening photo. Perform same as Option 2.

FIGURE 10.10 Flyes
(Pectorals; Anterior Deltoid)

OPTION 1: Floor Flyes

Position: Lie on your back, holding 1-lb – 4-lb hand weights in each hand above your shoulders, with your arms slightly bent (a).

Action: Inhale as you move weights away from each other and lower them toward the floor (b).

Action: Exhale as you return hand weights to starting position above you.

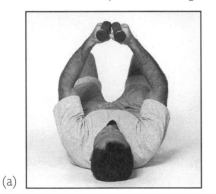

(a)

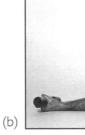

(b)

OPTION 2: Tubing and Aerobics

Position: Stand with bent knees, one heel forward and one foot back. Tube in front of chest, rolled up around your hands, for correct tube length (not shown).

Action: Pull hands horizontally apart (as wide as possible with resistance tubing you're using (c). Return to starting position, shifting weight and repeating with heel tap to opposite side.

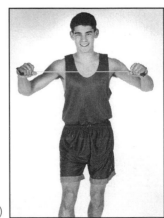

(c)

FIGURE 10.11   Chest (Pec) Cross-Over

Tubing   (Pectorals)

Position: Step on tubing with one or both feet, with slight bend in knees. Arms are away from body, in front of thighs, no tension.

Action: Cross arms at midline, wrists locked, elbows bent.

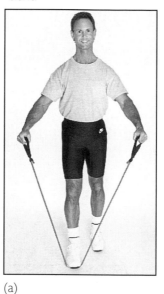

(a)

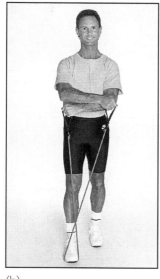

(b)

FIGURE 10.12   Seated Lat Row

Tubing   (Lats/Trapezius/Rear Deltoid)

Position:
Seated, with both knees bent, toes pointed forward, abdominals contracted (to protect lower back). Hands at waist level, fists facing, arms away from body.

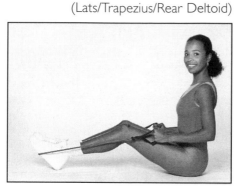

(a)

Action: Pull elbows behind body, fists facing sides; keep head and spine stationary.

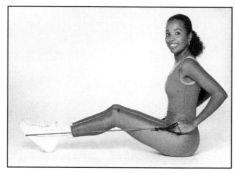

(b)

FIGURE 10.13   Lat Pull-Down

Rolled-up Tubing   (Latissimus Dorsi)

Position: Grasp band with R hand and place overhead. R elbow is slightly bent, and band is anchored above/behind center of your head.

Action: Grasp band with L hand, keeping hand away from L ear, slowly pull down so L elbow comes toward L side of body. Control the return.

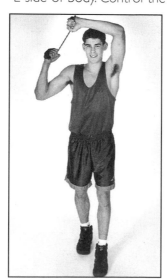

(a)

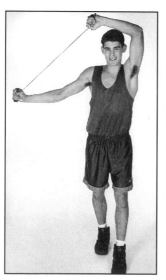

(b)

FIGURE 10.14   Deltoid Lateral Raise

(Deltoids/Trapezius)

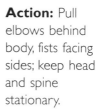

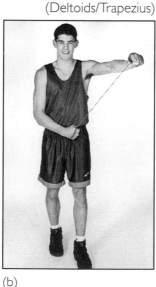

(a)   (b)

OPTION 1:   Rolled-Up Tubing

Position: Grasp band with L hand and anchor it on R hip/side/thigh. Grasp band with R hand, firm fist facing side, elbow bent.

Action: Pull slowly out wide to shoulder height.

(continued)

FIGURE 10.14 DELTOID LATERAL RAISE Continued

(Deltoids/Trapezius)

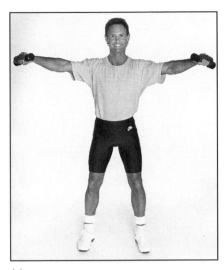

(c)

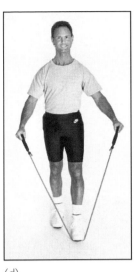

(d)

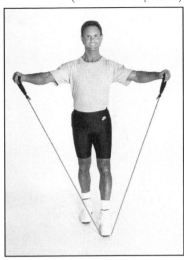

(e)

OPTION 2: 1-lb – 4-lb Hand Weights

Position: Standing astride, with hand weights resting on side of thighs.

Action: Raise one arm, or both together (c) to the shoulder-level position. Control the return.

OPTION 3: Tubing

Position: Step on tubing with R foot while L foot is behind and L of midline, knees and elbows slightly bent.

Action: Raise elbows away from sides up to shoulder level while keeping wrists/forearms locked, and hands slightly higher than elbows.

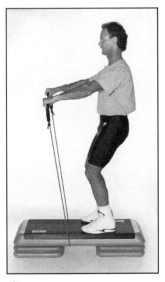

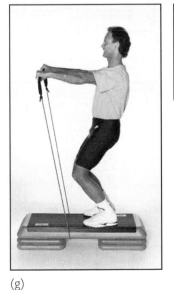

(f)

(g)

Note: Bent knees in some of these illustrations assist in keeping a target heart rate, so that these exercises also can serve as 1-minute strength-training "intervals" in aerobic step training with strength programs.

OPTION 4: With Squat

Bench and Tubing

Position: Stand on top of bench with tubing under center, having a fists top/thumbs in and down position.

Action: Press up, bending knees, with hands leading, going only to shoulder level or lower. If fatigued, raise arms just half way (h).

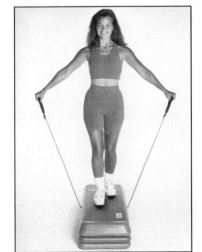

(h)

OPTION 5:

Without Squat

Bench and Tubing

Action: If fatigued, raise arms just half way.

FIGURE 10.15   Upright Row

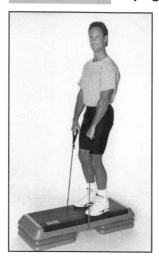

(a)

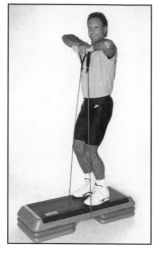

(b)

Bench and Tubing   (Deltoids/Trapezius)

Position: Initial foot and tubing position are the same, hands/fists now facing and resting on thighs.

Action: Raise handles up to chin, flaring out elbows slightly, keeping spine firmly erect.

OPTION:

Perform the upright row using just the tubing, without the bench.

FIGURE 10.16   Bicep Curls   (Bicep/Brachialis)

OPTION 1:

Tubing

Position: Step on tubing with one/two feet, slight bend in knees, and fists/palms facing body, wrists locked, elbows kept at sides throughout (a).

Action: Curl both arms toward shoulders (b).

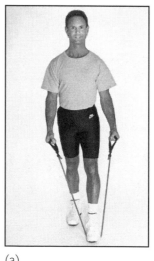

(a)

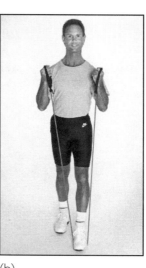

(b)

OPTION 2:

Double Tubing

– New idea –
(advanced)

Position: Same, except place both tubing handles in one hand (c).

Action: Curl arm with tubing (use other hand as a stabilizer).

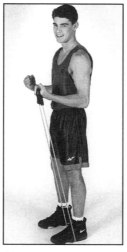

(c)

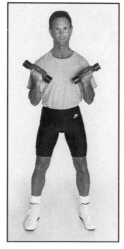

(d)

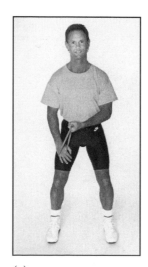

(e)

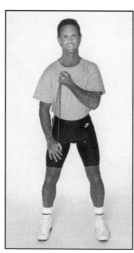

(f)

OPTION 3:

1-lb – 4-lb Hand Weights

Position: Resting weights near thighs, palms up.

Action: Raise one arm, or both together (d). If just one is used, alternate.

OPTION 4:   Band

Position: L hand anchors band on L thigh. Grasp band with R hand, keeping wrist locked, and R elbow against side (e).

Action: Curl up arm past chest, wrist ending center and toward R shoulder (f).

FIGURE 10.16 Bicep Curls Continued

OPTION 5: With Squat

Bench and Tubing   (Bicep/Brachialis)

Position: Same standing, tube location as in Upright Row, and hand/fist position facing thighs.

Action: Curl up to sky, rotating palms on the way up so they face shoulders. Reverse rotation for return. Bend knees to increase heart rate.

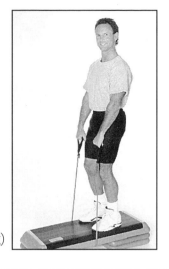
(g)

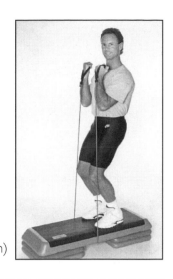
(h)

FIGURE 10.17 Triceps Kick (Press) Back   (Triceps)

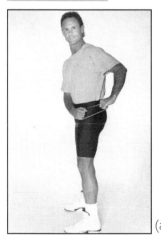
(a)

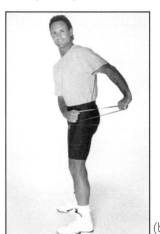
(b)

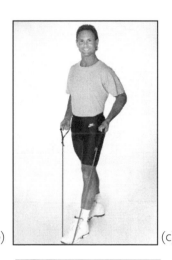
(c)

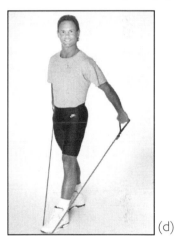
(d)

OPTION 1: Band

Position: Grasp band with L hand and anchor it on R thigh. Grasp band with R hand, palm/fist facing backward, relaxed position. L arm bent and stabilized against body.

Action: Press arm back to fully extended position.

OPTION 2: Rolled-up Tubing

Position: Place one handle in each hand and roll up tubing, until the length is about 1 foot (not shown). Repeat as shown in (a) and (b).

OPTION 3: Tubing

Position: Stand in forward/back stride position, grasp handles with palms facing up/in, elbows cocked.

Action: Press both arms backward, rotating wrists so palms are facing rear, firm wrists, arms fully extended.

FIGURE 10.18: Triceps Extension   (Triceps)

Tubing

Position: Stand on one handle with L foot. Grab other handle with L hand; grab the tube midway with R hand behind your back at the waist area. Raise L elbow, pointing skyward, lowering L hand to atop shoulder.

Action: Holding the tube firmly at the waist, extend L forearm skyward.

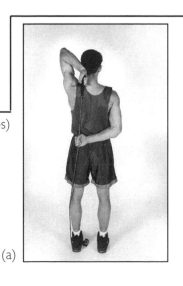
(a)

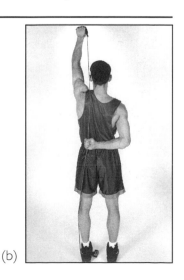
(b)

FIGURE 10.19   Overhead Press

(Deltoids/Triceps)

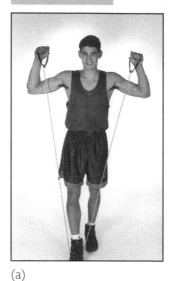

(a)

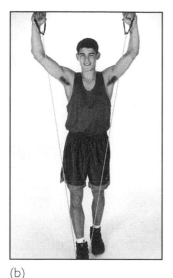

(b)

OPTION 1:   Tubing

Position: Stand with tubing under one foot; hands are holding tubing, with elbows shoulder high (a).

Action: Press upward to full extension, keeping elbows slightly flexed (b).

OPTION 3:   Tubing

Position: Sit on tube, bending knees, feet flat on the floor (c); continue as in (a) and (b).

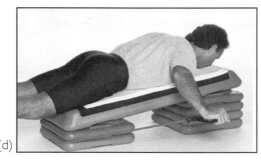

(c)

OPTION 2:   Incline Bench and Tubing

Adjust bench so two blocks are at low end and four blocks are at high end.

Position: Prone, with tubing in back of second block's groove, hands starting at sides, wide, and chin resting on incline bench top (d).

Action: Press up and forward, ending with thumbs in and facing each other (e).

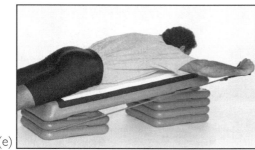

(d)

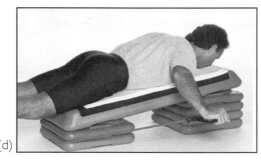

(e)

FIGURE 10.20   Back Extension

Incline Bench   (Erector Spinae)

Position: Lie prone with hips on lower third, legs extending off bench, supported by toes on floor. With chin on bench, place hands at hips area.

Action: Contract low back and raise upper chest; hands may move in a sliding motion backward. Lower.

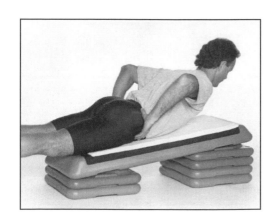

FIGURE 10.21   Curl-Ups   (Abdominals)

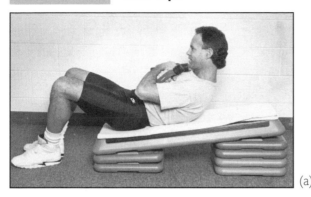

(a)

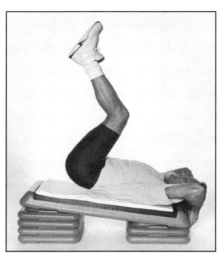

(b)

OPTION 1:   Gravity-Assisted Curl-Up

Incline Bench and 1-lb – 4-lb weights

Position: With bench in incline position, straddle and *sit on lower third.* Place a free weight* on sternum (breastbone), with knees flared out wide and heels together, flat on floor.

Action: Keeping lower back on bench at all times, curl up, head looking forward (a). This is all the farther you go; release and curl back down to lying position.

---

* Adding more weight resistance is optional, but if you do, this is where it should be done. Maximum hand weights to use on bench is 10 lbs.

OPTION 2:   Reverse Curl-Up

Decline Bench

Position: Place bench in a decline position, lie on bench, face up with *head at lower end* of bench. Grasp lip of platform and top block over your head. Legs are skyward, with hips, knees, and ankles bent softly.

Action: Contract abdominals and raise buttocks up, keeping lower back on the platform (b). Lower.

OPTION 3:   Curl-Up Variation

Position: Lie on your back, with fingers spread behind head, elbows wide. Bend L knee, with foot flat on floor; R leg lying on the floor.

Action: Keeping mid-to-low back on floor at all times, contract abdominals and curl up, head looking forward and up, while raising R leg to a thigh-parallel position (c). Lower head and R leg simultaneously. Repeat L leg.

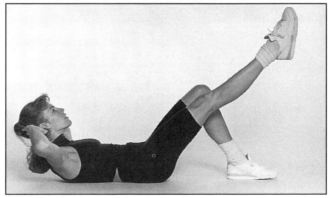

(c)

Note: Reps for abdominal work can be 15–30, and two sets — one *before* the aerobic segment and one *after* — because the type of muscle tissue located here responds better to more repetitions for definition than other groups of the body do. These exercises are to help strengthen sensitive lower back; the low back is completely supported during the abdominal contraction.

FIGURE 10.22   **Squats**   (Buttocks)

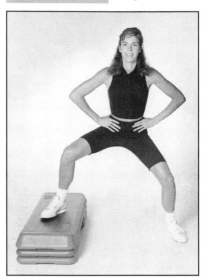

(a)

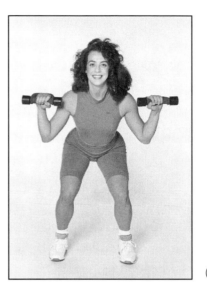

(b)

OPTION 1:   Bench

Position: Stand with your side next to side of bench. Place L foot on center of bench, R foot on floor in wide stance; hands on hips.

Action: "Wide-sit," flexing knees and lowering buttocks until knees are over, but not beyond, toes (a). Raise.

OPTION 2:   1-lb – 4-lb Hand Weights

Position: Stand with feet shoulder-width apart, holding 1-lb – 4-lb hand weights near shoulders, elbows at sides.

Action: "Sit," flexing knees and lowering buttocks until knees are over (but not beyond) toes (b). Raise.

FIGURE 10.23   Buttocks/Heel Lift

Band   (Gluteals)

Position: Assume an all-fours position, resting on forearms, knees wider than hips, abdominals tight. Place band around L ankle and R instep.

Action: Bend R leg with heel pointing to ceiling, lifting heel without bending knee any further, going as far as band will allow. Lower. Alternate legs to achieve balance.

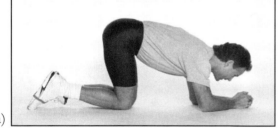

(a)

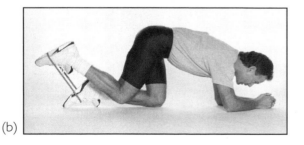

(b)

FIGURE 10.24   Side Leg Raise

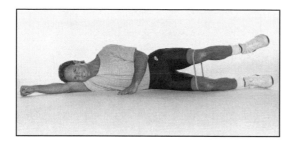

Band   (Thigh Abductors)

Position: Place band just above knees. Lie on side, with head resting on bottom arm, which is straight overhead. Top arm is in a bent-arm support in front of chest, with legs either slightly bent or knees bent to 90°.

Action: Raise top leg (bent as shown) 6"–12", toward ceiling. Control body position during raising and lowering. After reps, change position and alternate, to strengthen both legs.

FIGURE 10.25   Inner Thigh Lift

Band   (Thigh Adductors)

Position: Lie on side with band placed around instep of both feet. Cross top leg forward, over bottom leg, and place foot flat on floor.

Action: Lift bottom leg up toward ceiling as far as you can, with toes slightly higher than heel. Lower leg slowly, not allowing it to touch floor. After reps are completed, alternate legs.

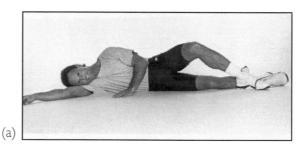
(a)

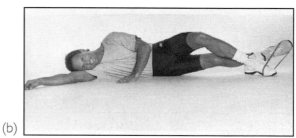
(b)

FIGURE 10.26   Leg Curl

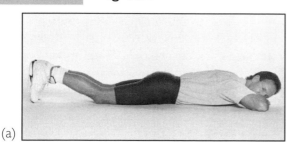
(a)

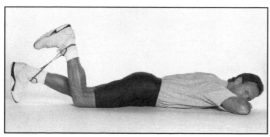
(b)

Band   (Hamstrings)

Position: Lie face down, with band around ankles.

Action: Bend R leg, bringing heel toward and within 12"–18" of buttocks, keeping hips down firmly on floor. Return. Alternate.

Note: An excellent exercise for the quadriceps, as a balance to this exercise, is shown in Figure 10.3. Hips again are held firmly on the floor, and the action is alternated after the reps, for balance.

FIGURE 10.27 Heel Raise with Squat

Bench and Tubing (Gastrocnemius/Soleus)

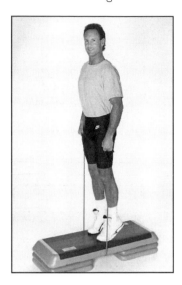

Position: Feet center, standing tall. Tubing is placed under center of bench and held at sides of hips.

Action: Keeping palms stationary (they do not move) at sides, raise heels up, contracting calves ("squeeze"). Lower back down and bend knees. Maintain excellent body alignment.

Seated Lower Leg Flexor and Extensor (see Figures 3.6–3.7)

Tubing (Anterior Tibialis)

Position: Sit tall, chest raised, shoulders down, holding handles near thighs, palms down, with tubing around ball/toe area of both feet held close together.

Action: Without moving body or hands, point toes away from you.

Action: Now, without moving body or hands, point toes toward you, flexing ankles. (This is a great exercise for prevention or relief of shin splints.)

Note: Securing the tubing firmly around toes while holding the tubing firmly in place will prevent it from rolling off your toes and toward your face/chest area for this exercise.

IMPLEMENTING AND RECORDING YOUR STRENGTH-TRAINING PROGRAM

Various equipment can be used to train the muscle groups, so whatever your preference or whatever is available to you, you have at least one way to strength-train each muscle group. Even while you are traveling, you can easily pack the light resistance bands or tubing and continue your program uninterrupted.

Recording your strength-training progress will prove to be a motivational tool for you to continue your program after the formal structure of a fitness class setting ends. Record the following in Figure 10.28, and then continue in a journal:

● The specific exercise techniques you choose for your program.

● The number of sets and reps of each exercise you perform.

● The types of weight resistance used.

● The date of the workout.

Begin the strength-training segment of your program slowly, methodically, and in absolute control of the amount of resistance or weights you are using. Strength-fitness training to develop muscle strength and endurance more fully is a long-term project.[14] It calls for a dedicated personal commitment of many hours, just as the programs of stretching for flexibility improvement and aerobics for aerobic capacity improvement are. All fitness programs are for life.

Even while you are traveling,
you can easily pack the light resistance bands and tubing
and continue your program uninterrupted.

FIGURE 10.28   Recording Form for Strength Training

Strength Training with Bands, Tubing, Light (1-lb – 4-lb) Free Weights and Tubing with the Bench							
Date							
Exercise	S / R / Res*	S / R / Res*	S / R / Res*	S / R / Res*	S / R / Res*	S / R / Res*	S / R / Res*

*S / R / Res = Sets, Repetitions, and Resistance (e.g., 3 / 8 / MT = 3 sets of 8 repetitions with medium tubing).

Goal Setting Challenge

Giving *definition* (shaping/toning/sculpting) to your muscles not only will make you look better but also will provide you with more strength and endurance to perform all of your daily tasks. These are two good reasons to set a goal to strength-train regularly, using your favorite resistance from the variety presented.

Developing Goal Scripts for Chapter 10

DIRECTIONS: Write complete sentences for each segment below. Combine your responses to all four segments. This goal script is designed around your needs and choices. Read it (or make an audiotape and play it) twice daily, morning and evening, until you master it.

❶ State one goal in positive, *present-tense* language. Ask yourself, "What will I experience — see, hear, taste, smell, feel — in regard to the results? Keep in mind that all powerful goals use the SMART formula: specific, measurable, achievable, realistic, timely.

_____

_____

❷ State your *pleasure-value reasons*. Ask yourself, "Why am I totally committed to achieving this goal? What am I choosing to feel?"

_____

_____

❸ State your *pain-avoidance value reasons*. Ask yourself, "What painful values do I choose to avoid feeling?"

_____

_____

❹ State *immediate action(s)* you can take in the next 24 hours. Use positive, present-tense verbs such as *choose* and verbs ending with "ing."

_____

_____

Cool-Down and Flexibility Training

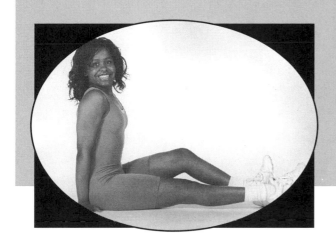

The final segment of a total fitness program consists of (a) the cool-down and (b) flexibility training. Because they are complementary, these two types of activity are presented together in this chapter.

COOL-DOWN

The purpose of a planned cool-down portion of your fitness session is to give your body time to readjust to the pre-activity state in which you began. This will ease the gradual process of returning the large quantity of blood now in your working muscles, primarily in your arms and legs, back toward your head and trunk, brain, and other vital organs.

Abruptly stopping a highly strenuous activity session may cause the blood (primarily in your legs) to pool or to stay in the extremities. This will occur because the veins of the legs are not being forcefully squeezed now by strenuously working leg muscles. The result of pooling can cause cramping, nausea, dizziness, and fainting, because the needed quantity of oxygen and blood is not being delivered to the brain and other vital organs.

Your ability to recover from exertion usually will determine how long your cool-down period will have to be. A minimum of 5 to 10 minutes is essential, however, for two reasons:

1. To curtail profuse sweating.

2. To lower the heart rate to below 120 beats per minute.

These are two visible signs to monitor and achieve before concluding your exercise session.

You'll begin your cooling-down process by slowing down all large muscle activity completely. Tapering off your activity level can be done in various ways, using lower intensity and lower impact moves that gradually decrease your heart rate.

The exercises are still active and rhythmic, using a full range of motion, but now are low-level and slower, half-the-tempo moves, with arms changing from big moves to decreasingly smaller type moves. Examples of cool-down moves are:

- pressing and lunging (Figure 11.1)
- two-foot bouncing, with a variety of mid/low arm gestures (Figure 11.2)
- a step tap (toe or heel) facing the bench using various directional approaches and arm gestures (Figure 11.3)
- wide-stride standing, upper- and lower-body strength conditioning moves (performed *without* weights) such as a squat with bicep curls (Figure 11.4); or
- slow-paced walking (Figure 11.5).

FIGURE 11.1

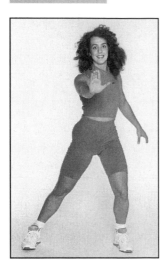

Pressing and lunging.

FIGURE 11.2

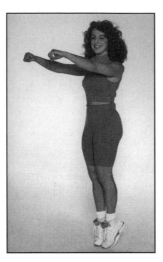

Two-foot bouncing.

FIGURE 11.3

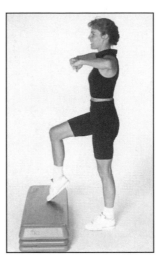

Step tap (toe or heel).

FIGURE 11.4

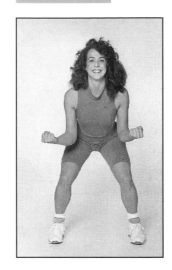

Squat and curls.

FIGURE 11.5

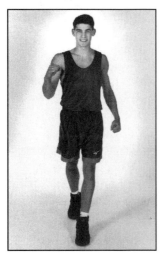

Slow-paced walking.

Research tells us that the highest incidence of problems occurs after an intense workout, so be sure to take this needed time (5 minutes minimum) to readjust.

Depending on whether you have just finished aerobic exercise or the optional strength-training segment, the time may vary as to how long this transitional cool-down will require. Give yourself time to readjust your pulse, breathing, and other physiologies. Research tells us that the highest incidence of problems occurs *after* an intense workout, so be sure to take this needed time (*5 minutes minimum*) to readjust. This segment begins the transition between the vigorous activity you've just completed and the flexibility training and relaxation you will perform last.

FLEXIBILITY TRAINING

Flexibility training, or stretching is a widely accepted means of effectively increasing joint mobility, improving exercise performance, and reducing injuries.[1] Flexibility refers to the range of motion of a joint and its corresponding muscle groups. It is influenced genetically, highly specific, and varies from joint to joint within an individual. When stretched repeatedly, muscle can be lengthened by approximately 20%,[2] and tendons can increase in length only about 2% to 3%.

Stretching programs follow the principle of specific adaptation to imposed demands (SAID), which states that an individual must slowly and progressively stretch the soft tissues around a joint to and slightly beyond the point of limitation but not to the point of tearing.

At present, the two most widely accepted methods of stretching to improve flexibility are static and proprioceptive neuromuscular facilitation (PNF). Both follow the philosophy that flexibility is increased and risk of injury is prevented when the muscle being stretched is as relaxed as possible.

Static Stretching

Static stretching is slow, active stretching, with the position held at the joint extremes. The aim is to *ease gently into a controlled, stretched position and hold it as you press gently* (Figure 11.6). You push

FIGURE 11.6   Static Stretching

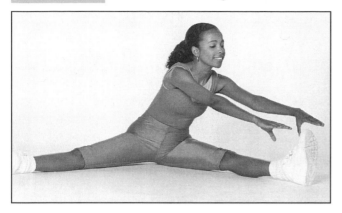

or press to the point of tightness, "stretch pull" (not a pain, but a tight feeling) so you feel the muscle working. You continue to stretch a little beyond this point, without any motion. Then, mentally, you relax your mind and hold the position for approximately 15 seconds, allowing the muscle to also relax and feel heavier.[3] Performing the same stretching on the opposite side of your body always follows.

At present, static stretching is considered one of the most effective methods of increasing flexibility. Research has shown that significant gains can be achieved with a training program of static stretching exercises. This type of continuous stretching produces greater flexibility with less possibility of injury, probably because it stretches the muscles under controlled conditions.

PNF Stretching

PNF stretching techniques, in which muscles are stretched progressively with intermittent isometric contractions, also offer an effective method of increasing flexibility and are used, like static stretches, when the muscles are warm. Two of the most commonly used modified PNF stretches are:

1. *Contract-relax technique:* In phase one, perform a 5–6 second maximum voluntary contraction in the muscle to be stretched. The contraction is isometric because any motion is resisted. In phase two, relax, then stretch, the previously contracted muscle.

2. *Agonist contract-relax technique:* In phase one, maximally contract the muscle opposite the muscle to be stretched against resistance (a

partner, the floor, or other immovable object) for 5–6 seconds. In phase two, relax the agonist muscle and stretch the antagonist muscle.[4]

An example of a forward PNF contract-relax exercise for the hamstrings and spinal extensors, shown in Figure 11.7, is performed with a partner's assistance.

FIGURE 11.7

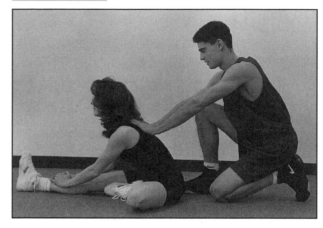

Forward PNF contract-relax stretching.

Position: In a modified hurdler stretch position the performing partner leans forward to the point of limitation while keeping the back straight and the toes of the extended leg facing upward to stretch the hamstrings correctly.

Action: To begin the action, the performer pushes her back against the partner (contracting the spinal extensors) and pushes the extended leg against the floor (contracting the hamstrings) for a 6-second isometric contraction. The partner resists any movement gently but firmly.

Action: Releasing the contraction, the performer stretches to a new point of limitation, holding a static stretch for 12 seconds or longer, while the partner maintains a light pressure on the performer's back.

Stretching Sequence (on floor)

Stretching to increase your flexibility and range of motion is crucial, at this point in your session. It is the time when your muscles are *warm* (full of blood, oxygen, and nutrients) and your joints are pliable from vigorous exercise, so take full advantage of the next 5 to 10 minutes to static (or PNF) stretch. Many stretching techniques are presented in Chapter 6 (Figures 6.2–6.14). Refer to any of them to incorporate into this flexibility training segment. Add the sitting and lying-down stretches sequenced and presented in Figures 11.8–11.15, some of which can be performed on the step bench.

FIGURE 11.8 Hips/Groin/Calves Stretch

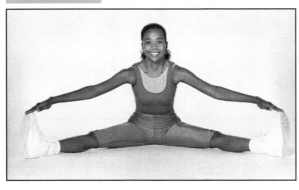

Position: Sit tall with your feet comfortably apart, arms shoulder high over legs, kneecaps and toes pointing skyward.

Action: Flex toes back toward you as you bend forward at hips, placing hands on shins/ankles/toes (whatever you can reach), leaning forward and stretching. Hold 8/16 counts. Relax and recover to start.

FIGURE 11.9 Groin/Hips Stretch

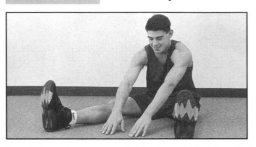

Position: See Figure 11.8. Then bring hands inside the "V."

Action: Lean forward from hips, and reach forward as far as you can, keeping head in line with spine. Hold 8/16 counts. Relax and recover to start.

FIGURE 11.10 Lower Back/Hamstrings Stretch

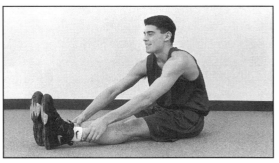

Position: See Figure 11.9. Then slide legs together, grab ankles/calves.

Action: Lean forward slowly from hips. Hold 8/16 counts. Relax and recover to start.

FIGURE 11.11 Lower Back/Hamstrings Stretch

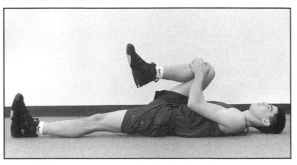

Position: See Figure 11.10. Now bend your knees, round your back, and lie down. Stretch long (not shown).

Action: Bring one knee up to chest, encircling it with hands. Pull knee to chest, keeping other leg long-stretched on floor, foot flexed. Hold 8/16 counts. Relax and recover to start. Repeat with other leg, 8/16 counts.

Stretching Sequence (on bench)

FIGURE 11.12   **Back Stretch**

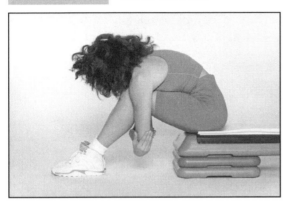

Place towel on bench. Sit on end of bench with your feet together on the floor. Bend over, resting your chest on thighs. Reach under legs with arms, grasp the opposite elbow, and pull both elbows together. Hold. 8/16 counts.

FIGURE 11.13   **Pectoral Stretch**

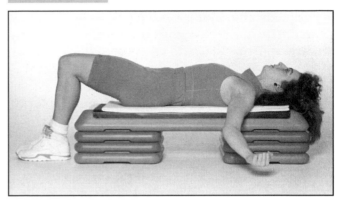

Lie down on platform with head and buttocks both comfortably on bench. Press low back into bench and place arms out wide to sides, shoulder level, and palms up. Relax arms as their weight falls toward the floor. Hold. 8/16 counts.

FIGURE 11.14   **Hamstring Stretch**

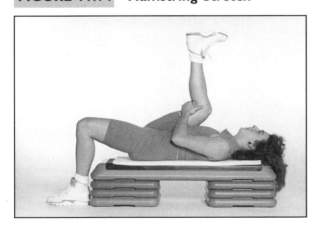

Lying on bench, extend L leg straight out along platform and place foot flat on floor. Grasp behind R thigh and gently pull R leg toward chest. Hold. *Ankle Stretch:* During the hamstring stretch, slowly circle the foot in all directions. Alternate with L leg and foot. 8/16 counts each.

FIGURE 11.15   **Achilles/Calf Stretch**

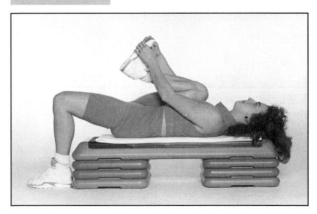

From the hamstring stretch (Figure 11.14), pull R knee to chest. Grasp R toes with hands and pull gently. Hold. Alternate with L leg and foot. 8/16 counts each.

STATIC STRETCHING WITH RELAXATION

At the conclusion of your workout, enjoy the natural high your endorphins are giving you, and begin relaxation techniques during the final stretching segment. This is an excellent time to develop rich images and affirmations for yourself (see Chapters 2 and 12), starting with your energized muscles now becoming "wider-and-longer-and-warmer-and heavier." Your breathing is sequential with the pictures and affirmations. Breathe in deeply for 8 counts, hold your breath, and exhale and stretch for 8/16 counts.

A complete program of relaxation techniques is presented in Chapter 12 to finalize your total physical fitness workout session.

FIGURE 11.16 **Lateral Neck Stretches**

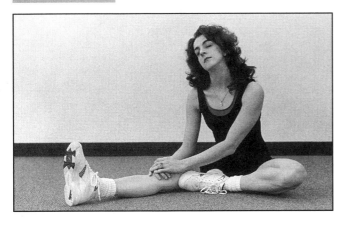

In half-hurdler position (sole of R foot against L inner thigh), drop head to L side. Hold 8/16 counts. Switch leg positions and drop head to R side. Hold 8/16 counts. Relax with images and self-talk throughout.

FIGURE 11.17
Stretching (Lower Back/Hamstrings)

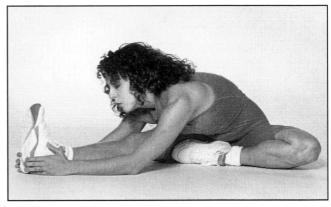

In half-hurdler position, lean forward, press, and hold 8/16 counts. Relax with images and self-talk.

FIGURE 11.18 **Relaxing on Step Bench**

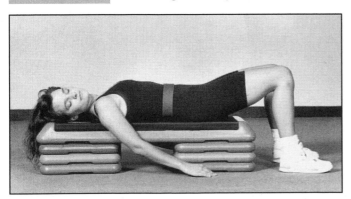

Continue relaxing, imaging, and self-talking when stretching is completed. These are the re-energizing moments of your session.

PROGRAM SEGMENTS IN REVIEW

Outlined below are the basic concepts of the four key segments of a total fitness program. Following a fitness program such as this will provide you with a fun, safe, efficient, and complete workout session. If you prioritize this type of total physical fitness program into your schedule, you will have an excellent means of initially obtaining and then maintaining your fitness for a lifetime.

SEGMENT 1: WARM-UP

- Active, rhythmic, limbering moves.
- Slow, standing, static stretching.
- Proper breathing technique throughout.

SEGMENT 2: AEROBICS/STEP TRAINING/ FITNESS WALKING

- Low-impact cardiovascular warm-up.
- Power low-impact with plyometrics.
- High- and low-impact.
- Power low-impact with plyometrics.
- Low-impact cool-down.
- Post-aerobic stretching.

SEGMENT 3: STRENGTH TRAINING

- Focusing on isolated muscle groups: chest, arms, abdominals, buttocks, thighs, shins, and calves.
- Adding hand weights, resistance bands, and resistance tubing.

SEGMENT 4: COOL-DOWN, FLEXIBILITY TRAINING, AND RELAXATION

- Gradual cool-down moves.
- Flexibility training using static and PNF stretching.
- Relaxation techniques during and after final stretching moves.

Goal Setting Challenge

Set several goals:
1. To stretch *every day* of your life for *5–10 minutes.*
2. To purchase a *daily planner* schedule book.
3. To *make a date with yourself* to work out consistently, regarding your Frequency, Intensity, and Time duration (your **FIT** formula), then *keep* every scheduled date with yourself!

Developing Goal Scripts for Chapter 11

DIRECTIONS: Write complete sentences for each segment below. Combine your responses to all four segments. This goal script is designed around your needs and choices. Read it (or make an audiotape and play it) twice daily, morning and evening, until you master it.

❶ State one goal in positive, *present-tense* language. Ask yourself, "What will I experience — see, hear, taste, smell, feel — in regard to the results? Keep in mind that all powerful goals use the SMART formula: specific, measurable, achievable, realistic, timely.

_____

_____

❷ State your *pleasure-value reasons.* Ask yourself, "Why am I totally committed to achieving this goal? What am I choosing to feel?"

_____

_____

❸ State your *pain-avoidance value reasons.* Ask yourself, "What painful values do I choose to avoid feeling?"

_____

_____

❹ State *immediate action(s)* you can take in the next 24 hours. Use positive, present-tense verbs such as *choose* and verbs ending with "ing."

_____

_____

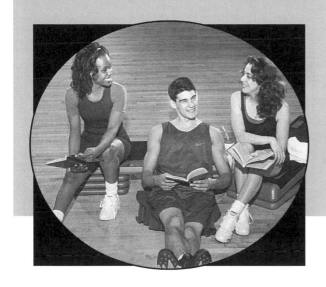

Stress Management and Relaxation

To the possession of the self,
the way is inward. —Plotinus

We each must, therefore,
"come of age" by ourself.
Each must journey to find our
true center, alone.

The physical training (workout) portion of your program is in place. Now is the time to reconsider the *mental* training aspects, to put completion to understanding how to establish a fitness program

To understand this final step requires you to make a decision. It's no "small choice" this time. It's time to make a leap-of-faith *commitment* to yourself *to be open to the possibilities available within you* and then have the courage to follow through and make the best choices from the knowledge you've gained thus far.

Therein lies the magnitude of the change you now are being asked to accept. The commitment you make requires *ownership* on your part (discussed in Chapter 2), *to keep the power to change.* By not blaming other people or things, you are empowered to use the creative potential within you. Your potential and answers are there. When you believe the creativity to problem-solve anything lies within you, *you find a way.* It simply needs to be awakened, called upon, and invited into action.

With this powerful thought fresh in your mind, set the goal-challenge for yourself now, *before* you get into this chapter. Committing yourself to being open to explore your creative potential is an exciting goal to set.

SETTING A STANDARD

Experiencing personal excellence in any or all of the dimensions of your life requires you to become more aware of your creative potential. To understand unlimited possibilities, we each must begin by setting a *standard* — establishing a starting point or basis — from which to grow. A balanced state of well-being (your stress in balance) expresses this ideal condition. By taking apart this abstract concept and labeling its parts, you will come to understand just how to initiate the process. This will lead to your managing the most productive and rewarding results imaginable in any and all of the dimensions of your life.

ESTABLISHING THE FOUNDATION

All of our world and universe is based on balance. Personal wellness is your life in balance. It requires actions, emotions, attitudes, beliefs, your will, and your power-source, all kept in mind and utilized in

Goal Setting Challenge

 Make a choice to update any thoughts you have that you cannot accomplish, improve, or master something. Ask yourself, "What is the biggest problem that I currently own?" — *something that up until now has eluded you.*

Can you then stretch your vision and goal-set to include the idea of becoming *a role model to others* in your fitness goal? Try it! You have everything to gain. Translate this powerful goal into a Goal Script *now*, on page 143.

solving problems. Life balance or *wellness* is illustrated in Figure 12.1 as six components or balls that we need to keep juggling in the air, all at once. These six components are: physical, emotional, social, spiritual, intellectual, and talent expression. Each of these components is an equally important contributor to the total balancing act we must engage in every day.

When any wellness component being juggled and kept in balance gets overlooked temporarily, or forgotten totally, it falls out of this balanced alignment and drops out of sight. We are then out of sync with life or get the feeling of not being whole. This is understandable because we aren't. We've allowed one component or several components of our lives to take over and receive all of our attention.

For example, if the expression of our talent (our job or career pursuit, or volunteering) takes an inordinate amount of our mental and physical energy every day, little time is left to participate in a physical fitness program, to develop a social network of friends, and to intellectually pursue other interests that can provide positive release of stress. Our physical, social, or intellectual ball drops. We soon experience the results — a decline in physical fitness, loss of a well-rounded social network of friends, or a boring, one-dimensional focus in our daily conversations.

SUCCESS

How do we know if and when we are truly balancing the six areas of our lives? Developing a working definition for *success* — knowing when you've achieved this balance — is one way. Take some quiet time to develop your own definition of success. Ask yourself, "What is balance in my life?"

Success is the ongoing process of striving and growing to become more, in each of the dimensions of wellness, while positively contributing to others' needs.

You can believe unconditionally that you are successful in anything you attempt in life if you (a) attempt and grow from it, (b) make more distinctions about what you're doing, and (c) accomplish it for the purpose of contributing positively what you've learned to others. By adopting this definition for success, it is difficult to feel like a loser or a failure.

Consider these points as steps in a journey rather than as a destination. Life is an ongoing process, and wellness and success are landmarks in the journey. Life has no one port or station — no one place to arrive at — once and for all. The true joy of life is the trip! A port or station evokes a mental image to be held in expectation so we can tap our unlimited potential in creative problem-solving. Life must be lived and enjoyed in the present moment as accomplished steps as we go along. The final port will come along soon enough.

BALANCING THE SIX WELLNESS DIMENSIONS

The *physical wellness* component is exemplified by a regular program of the physical expenditure of energy for increasing one's flexibility, heart and lung capacity, and muscular strength and endurance; maintaining a good posture while exerting this physical effort; selecting a proper intake of food and liquid; and maintaining the proper body weight.

FIGURE 12.1

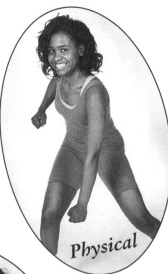

Physical

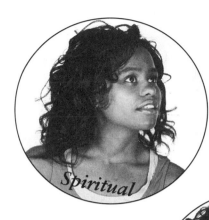

Spiritual

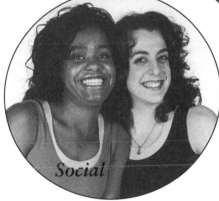

Social

Balance

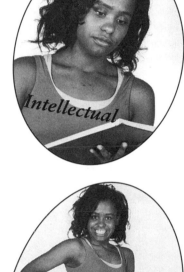

Intellectual

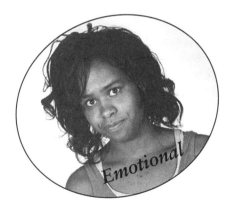

Emotional

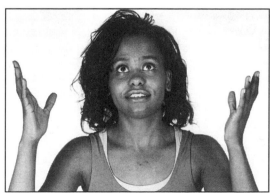

Talent Expression

Achieving wellness by balancing six key dimensions of your life.

The *emotional wellness* component deals with pleasure and pain (see Figure 12.2). It looks at the distinctions or labels for pleasure (joy) and pain (sadness, anger, fear) and the mixed neuro-associations we feel when these two driving forces are blended (confusion first, then an assortment and labeling of distinctive others). Becoming aware of the precise emotions we feel and what we *link* to pleasure and pain will assist us in being rational and able to choose productive behavioral responses to life situations.

The *social wellness* component involves creating balance in your time alone and time with others. Of course, we can choose to be independent and achieve every goal we ever set alone. You will discover, though, that the most successful and mature people, who tap into their full, unlimited potential regularly, are *inter*-dependent. They choose intentionally to interact with other people regularly even when they could fully accomplish their goals alone. They are able to stretch themselves to unbelievable heights because they draw constantly upon other people as their key resources.

Another theme in the social wellness component involves becoming aware of your communication skills. Sharpening your assertiveness and confrontational skills with others will assist you in becoming a victor instead of a victim in life.

The *intellectual wellness* component challenges you to become a lifelong learner, and to never become complacent and satisfied with past learning and accomplishments. Keeping an open mind to growth and change in the world at large will help us realize that our potential, individually and collectively, has no boundaries. The only boundaries or limits to our potential are the ones we self-impose inside our heads.

The *spiritual wellness* component challenges you to investigate the balance between relying on your own self-energy source (willpower) and that which ultimately fuels you. Finding purpose or the meaning of your existence is assisted by developing a belief system from your values. This is expressed as the philosophies by which you live your life daily, as you interact with others, the environment, and your inner self.

FIGURE 12.2

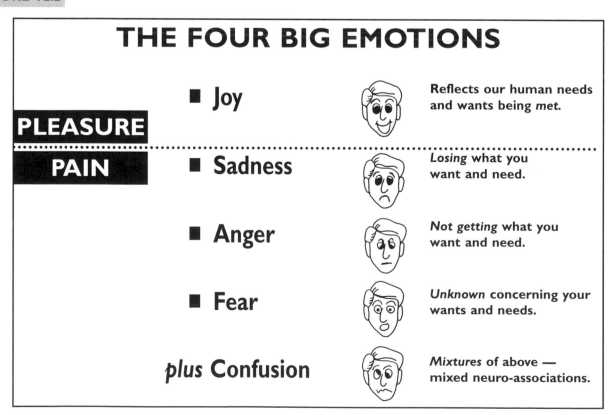

The four big emotions.

The *talent expression* component is the sixth dimension of wellness. Your talents are your natural and trained abilities and interests that become translated into your career path or jobs, the volunteer giving of your time to others, and many times the activities you engage in to relieve your stress (stress outlets). Because it usually has a significant impact on self-worth and prestige, this probably is one of the most difficult components for us to keep in perspective and balanced with the other five dimensions of wellness.

Why do we want to keep our wellness in balance — for what reasons, purposes, intentions? The five clearly defined survival *needs* we all must have met, supported by the wellness components of our lives, are:

1. I need to live and be healthy.
2. I need safety and security.
3. I need to be loved.
4. I need prestige (self-worth) and power (the ability to take action).
5. I need variety and change in my life.

These needs are *birthrights* that we all require for survival and never should be taken away or used as avenues by which to manipulate others.

In addition to our five basic needs are our wide variety of wants. Our *wants* are the privileges or extra comforts we attempt to attain by being responsible and accountable for the actions we take in life. We should begin to label not only what we require for survival (our *needs*, which we also call our ends or ultimate goals) but also what gives us additional pleasure and joy in the process (our *wants*, also called the means to our ends, or our time priorities). When we clearly understand both our basic needs and our desires or wants, we can pinpoint the purposes of and intentions for our various wellness decisions.

> *To reveal myself openly and honestly takes the rawest kind of courage.*[1]

The foundation of life is grounded in balance or a *wellness state*, composed of these six dimensions: physical, emotional, social, spiritual, intellectual, and talent expression.

> *The foundation of life is grounded in balance or a wellness state, composed of six dimensions: physical, emotional, social, spiritual, intellectual, and talent expression.*

DEFINING AND MANAGING STRESS

What happens when we become imbalanced and stress enters our life? We must be realistic and aware that life will not be a continual, perfect balance for us, because life is not static and unchanging. Change is a constant. Thus, we must consider how to deal with imbalance in our life.

Demands. Problems. Challenges. Change. Whatever you choose to call it, imbalance happens within the journey of life. We cannot control our world and all it presents to us. Drunk drivers injure us permanently. Fire and floods destroy our homes and belongings. Death takes our loved ones. A close friend moves far away. We win the lottery. Imbalance asserts itself daily and throughout our life, and we are left to react. *Stress* is our response. We cannot control the changes, demands, problems, or even the dirty deals we encounter, but we can learn how to manage certain situations so they are less offensive to us.

Probably the most noted scientific researcher in modern times on the topic of stress and its effect on the human body is the late Viennese-born endocrinologist Hans Selye. In his words: *Stress is the nonspecific response of the body to any kind of demand that is made upon it.*[2]

Selye established the groundwork on defining stress — which has been updated recently. Stress now is believed to be specific as a result of the scientific findings of the unique body of information called psychoneuroimmunology.

The new definition of stress is the following:

> *Stress: a series of positive or negative physiological responses and adaptations your body undergoes when any kind of demand is made upon it.*

Physiological Responses To Stress

The physiological response of your body to the positive or negative stressful demands impinging upon it from life situations includes:

● Increased sugar in the blood

- Increased rate of breathing
- Faster heart rate
- Higher blood pressure
- Activation of the blood-clotting mechanism to mitigate effects of injury
- Increased muscle tension
- Cessation of digestion, and diversion of blood to brain and muscles
- More perspiration output
- Decreased salivation
- Loosening of bladder and bowel muscles
- Outpouring of various hormones, including adrenalin
- Dilation of pupils of the eyes
- Heightening of all your senses.

In effect, your body goes into a "Red Alert" and you are ready to fight or flee. This has been aptly named the *fight or flight* response to stress.

Many times you can't do either — fight or flee. You must stay in the situation and "stew." If this response, as characterized by the above list, is long enough or severe enough, your bodily systems experience wear and tear. This leaves you open to the invasion of some sort of illness.

Once a person becomes ill, the illness also becomes a stressor. This increases your stress response (again, as described in the list of bodily changes) and you are caught in a double-bind.[3]

Good or bad, stress is our response to any kind of imbalance resulting from demands, problems, challenges, or changes. Therefore, scientifically and physiologically, stress is a neutral term. Positive stress, called *eustress*, is exemplified by running a marathon or seeing our loved one after 7 months of being away in the military. Negative stress, called *distress*, occurs, for example, when we are in a car accident or our home is vandalized. The goal in managing either kind of stress is the same as with all of life: to achieve a balanced state. This can be understood more easily using an analogy.

Stress management can be compared to playing a guitar. To play the guitar, we must use strings that come in a package, limp and with no tension on them (no demands or challenges). Without tension or stress on the strings, we can make no sounds. The same comparison goes for our lives. If we have no stress, we have no challenges, no risks, no growth. Life is boring, and so are we, because not enough is

going on in our life. But stretch those strings to their potential by placing them on the instrument with just the right amount of tension on them, add the human touch, and we will make beautiful sounds — harmony. Place too much tension on the strings (too many commitments on our time), and even the slightest pressure will cause the strings to pop — and so will we.

To experience life with continual growth, imbalance must occur to create room for new possibilities. Change is one of the certainties of life. It is a given. If we approach change from a positive perspective, it can open the doors to unlimited possibilities and growth. If we take the negative view and see it as a threat to our comfortable stability, change can imprison us in the depths of despair and result in stagnation. The choice of perspective, and our subsequent reactions, is ours to make.

Coping Skills

In the past, how have you chosen to use your resources to cope (regain balance) when life has dealt you an imbalancing experience? Have you begun to realize that to stay mentally balanced, we all do *something* to cope with the stress in our lives? Some of these coping mechanisms are positive, and some are negative and detrimental to our total well-being. How do you cope habitually with stress? What are your positive means, and what are your negative, detrimental means? Establish a goal to work on now, to improve the one response to stress that seems most disabling to you.

You probably will come away from this reflection a lot less judgmental of other people and their abilities to cope with stress. Knowing that we all do something to relieve and cope with the stress in our lives can help you tolerate another person's choices that sometimes affect you directly. You come away realizing that some people are not *bad* people because, say, they smoke cigarettes, but they simply are making a *bad choice* in coping with the stress in their lives.

Your success in adjusting to and managing your response to stress can provide you with growth and increased confidence to meet your next challenge (life situation). We each learn how to adjust to everyday big and small problems and life situations by using our vast internal resources. We are not born adjusted; we learn our adjustments systematically.

Guided Imagery

You can learn many effective strategies to manage stress. Developing your ability to relax is among the most important. Several guided imagery techniques are suggested to follow the positive stress of your workout session or to relieve the negative stresses you encounter every day. Each takes only a few minutes to visualize. If you use all of the techniques at one time, you will experience a *cumulative effect*, a deeper relaxation, perhaps even culminating in sleep.

Choose what result you desire. You may wish to simply enhance a workout with one brief relaxation technique lasting 3 minutes, to lower your heart rate and breathing, cease sweating profusely, and curb other physiologies. Or you may want to rejuvenate yourself for 10 minutes during a busy day by refocusing your attention before a big event such as an exam, speech, athletic contest, or interview, by using two techniques. At bedtime you may choose to relax totally to the point at which you go directly to sleep, which may entail using all of these techniques, plus others you develop.

In using these techniques, you might want to:

1. Have someone cue you by reading the steps slowly.
2. Record them slowly onto a cassette tape, then play them to relax.

Enjoy these classic guided-imagery techniques and then develop more imagery of your own. Take a "trip" to your favorite vacation spot or reexperience talking to the heroes and role models in your life.

*Ease the pounding of your heart
by the quieting of your mind.*

TOTAL BODY SCANNING

Total body scanning develops your life management skills through your imagination. Your mind seeks out and recognizes tension and eliminates it through your ability to imagine the relaxation. It requires no physical exertion or planned tensing of muscle groups. Total body scanning has four steps: (a) assuming the position, (b) establishing the breathing pattern, (c) tuning in to various parts of the body,

and (d) heart rate monitoring followed by simple static stretching to make you alert again (unless the technique is used prior to going to sleep).

Step 1: Assuming Relaxation Position

- Lie on your back. If you feel uncomfortable because your entire back is not in contact with the floor, raise one knee up with your foot flat on the floor approximately 1 foot from your buttocks (see Figure 12.3). Individuals with substantial buttocks or shoulder mass will find that this knee-up position will relieve the arched lower back feeling.

- Turn your head slightly to one side. When you become totally relaxed, your tongue will relax backward and cover your windpipe if you keep your head straight in line with the rest of you.

- Place your arms on the floor at your sides, palms down, with elbows slightly bent. Flexed joints are more relaxed.

- Place your legs apart (not crossed or in contact with one another). As the legs relax, your feet will tend to roll outward.

- If you relax best with your eyes open, keep them open. If you relax best with your eyes closed, close them. If you keep them open, focus continuously on one object only.

FIGURE 12.3 Relaxation Positions

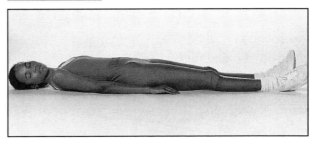

(a)

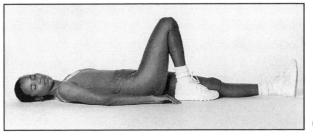

(b)

Step 2: Establishing Deep Breathing Pattern

- Take a deep breath and hold it in your lungs. Focus on the stretched-tight feeling you get in your chest by holding in the oxygen.

- Now, slowly and purposefully, breathe out (through puckered lips), a long, steady exhale. Create an image in your mind to lengthen the exhale. For example, see yourself blowing the fuzzy seeds off a dandelion that has gone to seed or blowing a long, steady note on a flute.

- Repeat this inhale, holding it, and follow with another slow, steady, long exhale. During this inhalation and exhalation, recognize that these next few minutes belong only to you. Do not share them with anybody or anything. Whatever problems, worries, or cares you have, including whatever you are going to do next in your day, briefly think what they are and list them all by writing them on a mental chalkboard in your mind. Then, again mentally, take out a big chalk eraser and wipe off each of them, one at a time, so you are looking at a blank chalkboard in your mind. Verbalize a thought to yourself (e.g., "This is my time now, and you [problem] are just going to have to wait"). Then forget it during your relaxation technique!

- Now follow your breathing cycle, whether it is fast, slow, regular, or irregular. Mentally tune in and follow each inhale and each exhale. Picture yourself on an elevator on which each exhale is a ride down one more floor (each inhale is the brief pause for the floor stop, door opening and closing). Or imagine that your mind is on a slow roller coaster ride of up and down, up and down.

- Don't interfere with your inhalation and exhalation. As you begin to relax, the exhalation (breathing out) becomes longer and longer. Ride with it and experience the longer ride out. This begins true relaxation.

- At various times during the entire body scanning relaxation technique, you will have to tune back in mentally to your breathing technique, for mastering this "elevator ride" is the central focus of your relaxation.

Step 3: Tuning In

- Start at the top of your head, travel down to the tips of your toes, and return to your mid-section.

- On the top of your head, mentally feel the "part" of your hair. Make it wide by relaxing your scalp.

- Mentally envision your ears. Drop all tension to your ears. If you are wearing earrings, mentally feel them as heavy on your earlobes.

- Tune in to your forehead. Is it tense and full of wrinkles? Make it flat and wide with no wrinkles. Picture it smooth.

- What is the space between your eyebrows doing? Is it grooved and full of wrinkles? Relax. Make a wide space between your eyebrows. This is one of the telltale locations of human stress. A person who is highly stressed seems to permanently tense the space between the eyebrows (contracted, wrinkled). Calm, serene people stand out because this small space is wide, relaxed, and untensed.

- Relax your eyebrows as if heavy weights were pulling down the ends. This also will relax your temple area.

- A hinge joint near your ear opening regulates your lower jaw. Relax that mandible joint by dropping your lower jaw. It will make your lips part. Relax your chin.

- When you relax your jaw, mentally feel your teeth and tongue. When some people try to practice total relaxation, they press (tense) their tongue tightly to the roof of their mouth. Also, many people grit or grind their teeth at night, an audible sign of tension.

- Relax your throat by thinking of the feeling you get with the second stage of swallowing. People who sing or play wind instruments have been trained in this technique to relax the area so the best sounds will come out of a relaxed vocal mechanism.

- Drop your shoulders and chest to make a wide space between your ears and shoulders. We unconsciously tense this area throughout the day. Whether we drive a car or walk in miserable weather, we tense the shoulders up near our ears, encouraging neckaches and headaches. When you think about it next time, untense these muscles.

- Allow the weight of your chest to sink through to the floor. Think "heavy chest."

- Drop all tension from your upper arms, elbows, lower arms, and hands until you can just feel your fingertips pulsating on the floor. You may feel a tingling in your fingertips.

- Relax your buttocks. This is the key to untensing the lower half of your body.

- Relax your kneecaps. This joint connects your upper and lower leg, and many times we tense the knee area when we attempt to relax other body parts. When you relax the knees, the upper legs will relax and the heavy weight of your legs will begin to drop to the floor. Likewise, the lower legs respond almost automatically, with the feet rolling outward.

- Mentally feel what your toes are doing. Are they tensed and curled under? If so, stretch them out and then relax them.

- Now return to the most difficult place to relax — the stomach and intestinal area. Focus your mind on the navel area and picture a wide, flat, picturesque pond. Envision a small pebble being tossed into the very center, creating a soft, rippling effect in which each ripple is a wave of relaxation. Feel the weight of your navel area sinking through, past your spine, onto the floor below you.

- Return to your breathing cycle, and follow it several times. Focus totally on the long, slow exhale.

- Now just rest a few moments and enjoy the totally untensed feeling.

Step 4: Heart Rate Monitoring and Stretching

- In the lying-down position, feel for your pulse. Mentally picture and feel your heart beating. Try to slow it down with your mind. Cue it to beat slower.

- Count your pulse for 15 seconds and multiply by 4 for a minute heart rate. How does this compare with your resting heart rate after 6–8 hours of sleep? What does 3 minutes of relaxation do for your body's recovery from exercise or daily stress?

- Before you get up, sit up slowly and stretch your arms, legs, chest, and back, so you become alert immediately (Figure 12.4). You must do this 15-second stretch or you'll find yourself yawning for an hour afterward! Of course, if you do this relaxation procedure before going to bed, omit this stretch.

FIGURE 12.4

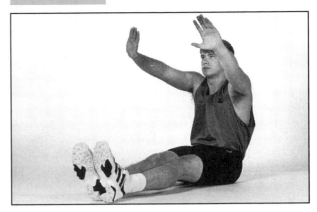

Sitting up slowly and stretching.

THE CONTROL PANEL WITH ONE LARGE DIAL

This second guided imagery technique has been found to be one of the easiest to visualize and integrate into a personal fitness program involving change. The control panel (Figure 12.5) is used now for rating, or quantifying, levels of tension and relaxation you feel within your body.

First, give a concrete label to each number on the control panel, from 0–10, as to what that level of relaxation/tension represents to you. Maybe 0 represents totally relaxed inner peace or lying on a warm beach, 5 represents balance and peak performances, and 10 means totally out of control or experiencing death, disease, or divorce. Write entries for what each number represents to you. Then give today's best/worst moments a number. Now that you have the idea of *quantifying stress*, visualize this second guided imagery technique.

- Visualize yourself in a safe place that represents relaxation to you, possibly your bedroom. Envision yourself there, seated in front of a control panel that has one large dial.[4] Continue to hold onto that image in your mind's eye for the duration of the technique, and soon you will feel as if you were actually there.

- Turn the dial to any setting from 0 to 10, which represents all the levels of relaxation and tension you are able to experience. Zero represents all of the relaxation that's possible for you to feel, and 10 represents as much tension as you are able to feel at one time.

- Begin to look closely at this dial that directly monitors and controls the level of tension in

FIGURE 12.5 Control Panel

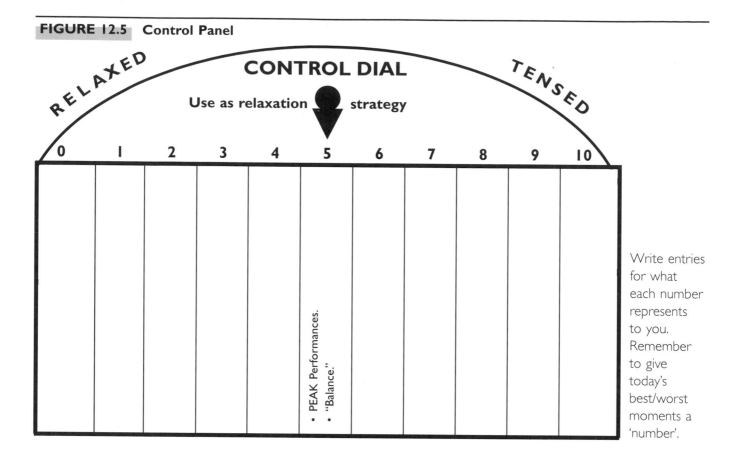

RELAXED

CONTROL DIAL
Use as relaxation strategy

TENSED

0 1 2 3 4 5 6 7 8 9 10

- PEAK Performances.
- "Balance."

Write entries for what each number represents to you. Remember to give today's best/worst moments a 'number'.

your body. What is the reading on the dial at this moment (from 0 to 10)?

- See yourself reaching over to turn it down. See yourself turning that dial down, v-e-r-y s-l-o-w-l-y, a little bit at a time. Feel your body relaxing more and more as you turn it down.

- Feel the tension in your body lessening more and more as you turn the dial all the way down. As all of the tension in your body ebbs away, turn the dial all the way down to zero. Your entire body is just as relaxed as it possibly can be. All of your previous tension is replaced with peaceful feelings of total relaxation and a centered calmness. Currents of gentle tranquillity soothe every muscle, every nerve, every fiber of your being.

- Return now to the moment in your day and the location where you were prior to your relaxation. Open your eyes and enjoy a fresh, new beginning.

From now on, relax just like this, whenever you choose, by sitting or lying down, closing your eyes for a few moments, and visualizing yourself turning down the dial on this control panel. The more you

practice this new ability, the more easily and the more deeply you'll be able to relax, and the longer these feelings of relaxation will remain with you.

You'll be able to sleep better at night, awaken more refreshed, work more efficiently without being bothered by people or situations during the day, feel rejuvenated to perform your very best when you need to, and enjoy your leisure-time activities to the fullest. Your unlimited potential awaits you in every aspect of your life. Whether it be rest, work, or leisure, every aspect of your life will be improved and enriched considerably by your new ability to relax whenever you choose.

NATURAL HIGHS

Natural highs are experiences that most likely made you feel good in the past. Relax, close your eyes, and take a long moment to remember the best times you ever had, experiencing each one of these.

Now create a list of your personalized natural highs from your own resources. First write them down, and then record them on a cassette tape. Whenever your stress is out of control, regain balance by listening to your own natural highs.

Natural highs . . . A fun new hobby. Swimming the last lap. Singing camp songs. A long distance call from a friend. Good grades. Water-skiing. A favorite hug. Your team winning. Listening to a friend giggle. Watching a sunset. Deciding not to watch your favorite TV show to get work done, and then finding out, after you finish, that your show was delayed and you still get to watch it. Your heart beat when you see someone you like.

Watching an animal take a bath in a patch of sun. Intercepting a pass. New pencils and supplies on the first day of school. Eating pizza with the works. A long, hot shower. Finishing a 10-K road race. A spider web with dew on it in the early morning sun. A great book. Reading under an electric blanket on a rainy day. Your first solo bike ride. International travel. Chili dogs. Reading before-and-after ads about overweight people. Intimacy. A good talk with a friend. A great idea. Snowskiing. A puppy.

Enthusiastic people. Climbing trees. God. Watching the moon. Plunging your hot body into a cool pool. Zoo animals nuzzling each other. An African violet that blooms. Running in the fall. Relaxing to Saturday morning cartoons. Making somebody laugh. Surfing. Walking on the beach. Decorating a Christmas tree. Playing the piano. Sailing. Fixing something that's been broken. Writing something exactly the way it has to be written to say what it has to say. A job well done. Creativity. Watching your favorite hockey team win in OT. Slumber parties. Meditation.

Liking your parents. The quiet after a snowfall. Riding down the street in a sports car switching gears. College friends. Singing in the shower. Cooking a favorite meal for friends. Really observing things. A letter from a friend. Seeing a rainbow after a shower. Being appreciated. Needlework. Losing fat weight. Being noticed by somebody you've been noticing. A warm inviting smile from a stranger. Success stories. Dancing.

Finishing a term paper. The first week of college. The last week of college. The day the yearbook came out. Uncontrollable laughter. Recognizing the truth in something you read. Hearing somebody say, "I love you." Holding hands. Clean hair. Stopping smoking. Stopping drugs. The first spring flower. Loving yourself. Breakfast in bed. Winks. A compassionate touch. . .[5]

YOUR OWN TIME-TUNNEL AND LOCATION FOR HANDLING EVERYDAY STRESS

Get yourself in a comfortable position, either sitting down comfortably or lying down, and make yourself relax as much as you can. And perhaps you'll close your eyes. And with your eyes closed, just roll your eyeballs up, as though you were looking right up through a spot on the inside of your forehead way up to the top of your head, and notice how much stress this puts on your eyes.

Now relax them, and notice how comfortable this feels by comparison. Let that comfort and relaxation spread to your jaw, so it hangs slightly open. Let it spread over your head, neck, shoulders, out into your arms, forearms, hands, fingers.

Take a deep breath, and feel the tension build up as you hold it, while I count one — two — three — four — five — now exhale . . . and notice how relaxing it is to exhale. And let this relaxation spread throughout your chest and into your abdomen, and into your hips, thighs, and all the way down to your feet and toes. Step into your own private time-tunnel . . . and transport yourself to a time when you were completely comfortable . . . no matter how long ago that might have been. Or if you prefer, you can travel into the future, to a more comfortable time that you can imagine than you can remember from the past.

And when you step from the time-tunnel, you can find yourself in a special place. It can be a real place or an imaginary place. A place you've been before or one you'd like to visit. Indoors or outdoors or any combination of these. The place can change with your mood, or the moment. And when you remember the comfortable feeling, close the hand you write with, gently into a fist, and reexperience those comfortable feelings over again, as you enjoy your special place . . . with all of your senses.

See the beauty of it. Notice the details . . . the colors . . . the lighting . . . the shadows . . . Notice who, if anyone, is there with you. Notice what is overheard . . . and overhead . . . and around you. Hear the sounds. . . Or if it is a quiet place, enjoy the silence . . . . Smell the fragrances . . . perhaps a special flower, or perfume . . . . Or maybe even a favorite food cooking . . . . Perhaps you can even taste it . . . . Most important, feel the comfort . . . .

And because this place is your own mental creation at this moment, the temperature should be perfect. It can be any kind of weather . . . any season of the year . . . and you can come to this place any time it is appropriate to do so . . . simply by closing the hand you write with and remembering how you feel, right now. . .[6]

Creating Your Own Guided Imagery

BEGIN BY:
- Finding a comfortable position.
- Closing your eyes.
- Focusing on your physical sensations.
- Practicing deep breathing.

NOW:

1. Pay attention to whatever tension-producing problem occurs to you at this moment. Put it into question form: " _____?"

2. Close your eyes and let your imagination *answer* the question you just asked yourself . . . .

3. Imagine *various* locations (beach/woods/mountains/your home or bedroom), and a season of the year (spring/summer/fall/winter).

   From these scenes and seasons, choose a place to relax that is uniquely satisfying to you:_____

4. Consider:
   - What does it smell like?_____
   - What are the sounds you hear? _____
   - What are the textures you feel? _____
   - What parts of you are moving, and how? _____
   - What do you see? _____
   - What are you saying when you talk to yourself?_____
   - What emotion do you feel in your body? _____

5. Imagine doing a relaxing activity such as:
   - Fishing/Lying on a warm, sandy beach
   - Enjoying a pleasant meal
   - Conversing with good friends
   - Sitting by a fire with a good book   • or: _____

6. By the time you have settled into your scene and relaxed in your imagination, your aches and pains, problem, or tension will soon be gone. Realize how powerful your imagination is, and can become. . .

LAST: Begin writing out your own guided imagery below. Think it out slowly and completely. Remember to use all of your sensual modalities (visual, auditory, kinesthetic, taste, smell) and as many submodalities as possible. (Submodalities describe the senses with detailed adjectives or adverbs, i.e., clear/loud/fuzzy/sweet/fragrant/fast, etc.).

OPTIONAL: Tape-record your guided imagery and use it to relax when needed.

_____

_____

_____

_____

_____

_____

_____

_____

_____

_____

Goal Setting Challenge *(from page 132)*

Ask yourself, "What is the biggest problem I currently own?" — something that up until now has eluded you. Set a goal below to master this challenge!

Developing Goal Scripts *before Chapter 12*

DIRECTIONS: Write complete sentences for each segment below. Combine your responses to all four segments. This goal script is designed around your needs and choices. Read it (or make an audiotape and play it) twice daily, morning and evening, until you master it.

1 State one goal in positive, *present-tense* language. Ask yourself, "What will I experience — see, hear, taste, smell, feel — in regard to the results? Keep in mind that all powerful goals use the SMART formula: specific, measurable, achievable, realistic, timely.

_____

_____

2 State your *pleasure-value reasons*. Ask yourself, "Why am I totally committed to achieving this goal? What am I choosing to feel?"

_____

_____

3 State your *pain-avoidance value reasons*. Ask yourself, "What painful values do I choose to avoid feeling?"

_____

_____

4 State *immediate action(s)* you can take in the next 24 hours. Use positive, present-tense verbs such as *choose* and verbs ending with "ing."

_____

_____

Goal Setting Challenge

Set a goal regarding how to manage your stress, the positive outlets you now choose to use, or regular time set aside to practice specific relaxation techniques. These are goals you'll not only enjoy setting but also experiencing how helpful they can be for the rest of your fitness program.

Developing Goal Scripts for Chapter 12

DIRECTIONS: Write complete sentences for each segment below. Combine your responses to all four segments. This goal script is designed around your needs and choices. Read it (or make an audiotape and play it) twice daily, morning and evening, until you master it.

1 State one goal in positive, *present-tense* language. Ask yourself, "What will I experience — see, hear, taste, smell, feel — in regard to the results? Keep in mind that all powerful goals use the SMART formula: specific, measurable, achievable, realistic, timely.

_____

_____

2 State your *pleasure-value reasons*. Ask yourself, "Why am I totally committed to achieving this goal? What am I choosing to feel?"

_____

_____

3 State your *pain-avoidance value reasons*. Ask yourself, "What painful values do I choose to avoid feeling?"

_____

_____

4 State *immediate action(s)* you can take in the next 24 hours. Use positive, present-tense verbs such as *choose* and verbs ending with "ing."

_____

_____

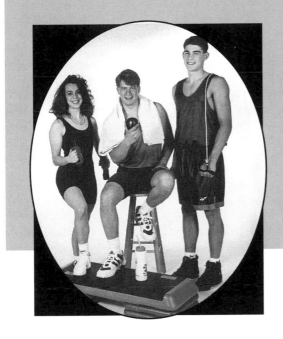

Nutrition

Choose what is best; habit will soon render it agreeable and easy.

Ancient philosopher Pythagoras stated this principle of making choices many years ago, and it hasn't really changed today. Better or best choices are always available for you to make. The actions you take reflect whether you simply have the knowledge or whether you *apply* the knowledge. Enjoy making the best available choices, all day long.

EATING FOR FITNESS

Your body needs two basic types of nutrients:

1. Foods that satisfy your energy needs.
2. Foods that meet your needs for growth, repair, and regulation of body processes.

Nutrients are chemical substances that your body absorbs from food during digestion. Your body needs at least 40 nutrients. *Diet* here means *total intake of food and drink*. Essential nutrients are those your body cannot make or is unable to make in adequate amounts. These nutrients must be obtained from what you eat and drink. If your diet does not provide them properly, your body cannot perform well, mentally or physically.

This is where choice comes in. You may know what the better choices of foods are (called *nutrient-dense* foods[1]), but if you don't eat the best choices

available to you, you really don't know good nutrition at all. Good health, optimum fitness, and good nutrition result from not just knowing what is best but actually choosing it 80% to 90% of the time.[2]

A well-balanced diet is one that contains these six basic nutrients:

1. Carbohydrates
2. Fats
3. Proteins
4. Vitamins
5. Minerals
6. Water

Proper amounts of each are established according to your age, gender, activity level, and state of wellness. These nutrients can be supplied from eating plans such as those presented here:

- Food Guide Pyramid. A Guide to Daily Food Choices, established by the U.S. Department of Agriculture[3] and shown in Figure 13.1, depicting the five major food groups;
- Pyramid Plus. A Star-Studded Guide to Food Choices for Better Health,[4] published by the Oregon Dairy Council, listing nutrient density information throughout the chapter and shown in Figure 13.3, depicting the number and size of servings recommended.

FIGURE 13.1 Food Guide Pyramid

Food Guide Pyramid
A Guide to Daily Food Choices

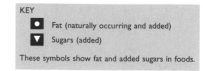

KEY

◻️● Fat (naturally occurring and added)
◻️▼ Sugars (added)

These symbols show fat and added sugars in foods.

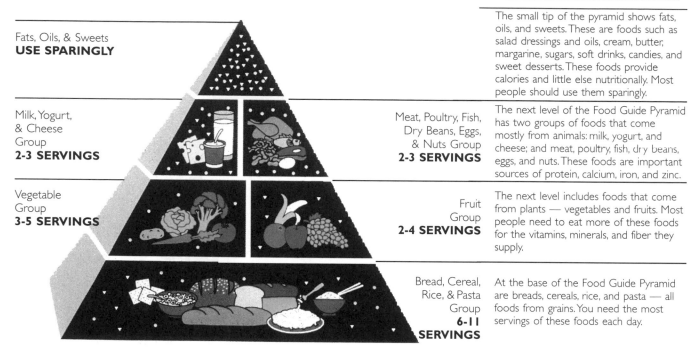

Fats, Oils, & Sweets
USE SPARINGLY

Milk, Yogurt,
& Cheese
Group
2-3 SERVINGS

Vegetable
Group
3-5 SERVINGS

Meat, Poultry, Fish,
Dry Beans, Eggs,
& Nuts Group
2-3 SERVINGS

Fruit
Group
2-4 SERVINGS

Bread, Cereal,
Rice, & Pasta
Group
**6-11
SERVINGS**

The small tip of the pyramid shows fats, oils, and sweets. These are foods such as salad dressings and oils, cream, butter, margarine, sugars, soft drinks, candies, and sweet desserts. These foods provide calories and little else nutritionally. Most people should use them sparingly.

The next level of the Food Guide Pyramid has two groups of foods that come mostly from animals: milk, yogurt, and cheese; and meat, poultry, fish, dry beans, eggs, and nuts. These foods are important sources of protein, calcium, iron, and zinc.

The next level includes foods that come from plants — vegetables and fruits. Most people need to eat more of these foods for the vitamins, minerals, and fiber they supply.

At the base of the Food Guide Pyramid are breads, cereals, rice, and pasta — all foods from grains. You need the most servings of these foods each day.

Source: From U.S. Department of Agriculture[3]

You cannot always take in all of the essential nutrients every 24 hours. What *is* important is that over a span of several days and weeks, you continually select from the five groups to meet your nutrient needs.

The pyramid is an *outline* of what to eat each day. It's not a rigid prescription but, rather, a general guide that lets you choose a healthful diet that's right for you. The pyramid calls for eating a variety of foods to get the nutrients you need and at the same time the proper amount of calories to maintain a healthy weight. The pyramid also focuses on fat because most American diets are too high in fat, especially saturated fat.

The pyramid emphasizes foods from the five major food groups shown in the three lower sections of the pyramid. Each of these food groups provides some, but not all, of the nutrients you need. Foods in one group can't replace those in another. No one food group is more important than another. For good health, you need them all.

Nutrient Density

Following the description of each food group, next, foods are listed according to *nutrient density, the amount of nutrition per calorie each food provides.* To get the most nutrition for the least calories, choose foods from the four-star groups (Figure 13.2), which are ranked *within* each starred group and listed in descending order of nutrients per calorie.[5]

The categories are:[6]

4 stars = most nutrition per calorie
3 stars = next to most nutrition per calorie
2 stars = next to least nutrition per calorie
1 star = least nutrition per calorie.

MILK AND MILK PRODUCTS GROUP

Calcium, riboflavin (vitamin B$_2$), and protein are the key nutrients needed to build the basic structure and strength of bones and teeth, assist in the production

FIGURE 13.2

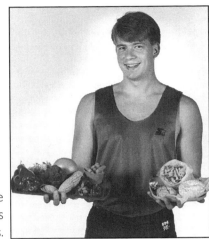

Nutrient-dense foods versus *calorie*-dense foods.

of energy needs, and help in the growth and maintenance of every living cell. If you are not an avid milk fan, you can eat other foods in the milk and milk products group (Table 13.1), and they will supply the calcium, riboflavin, and protein you need.

MEAT AND MEAT ALTERNATIVES GROUP

Key nutrients are *iron, protein,* niacin, thiamin, zinc, and B$_{12}$. Even though this group is called the "meat group," plant foods, when eaten together, can supply the needed protein, niacin, iron, and thiamine and are considered an alternative to eating meat (Table 13.2). Some of the plant foods that can be combined so their proteins complement each other (allow the amino acids to combine to form balanced protein) are: dried beans and whole wheat, dried beans and corn or rice, peanuts and wheat.[7]

One serving is equal to 2-3 ounces of cooked lean meat, fish, or poultry, or the protein equivalent. Visually, a 2- to 3-ounce portion fills the palm of an average hand and is the width of the little finger. All excess fat should be removed from any meat you eat. You should remove the skin from poultry and eat only the meat, eliminating unnecessary calories.

TABLE 13.1 Ratings of Milk and Milk Products

Rating:	Food Choices in Ranked Order for Calcium
	nonfat plain yogurt, nonfat milk nonfat cream cheese 1% milk buttermilk lowfat cheese 2% milk
	part-skim ricotta cheese whole milk regular fat cheese lowfat chocolate milk lowfat fruit yogurt nonfat frozen yogurt
	pudding custard lowfat frozen yogurt ice milk
	milkshake cottage cheese ice cream nonfat sour cream

TABLE 13.2 Ratings of Meat and Meat Alternatives

Rating:	Food Choices in Ranked Order for Iron and Protein
	fish, shellfish poultry (light meat, skinless) turkey ham beef (round and sirloin, well-trimmed) pork (tenderloin, well-trimmed) veal (leg and shoulder, well-trimmed) lentils
	beef (rib, chuck, flank and ground) ham (lean), tofu veal and lamb (leg and loin) poultry (dark meat with skin) pork (loin and rib) Canadian bacon poultry sausage dried beans and peas eggs
	hot dogs pork sausage chicken nuggets fish sticks nuts and seeds
	peanut butter bologna

VEGETABLE GROUP

Key nutrients are *folic acid, Vitamins A and C*, which are catalysts or action starters, and fiber (Table 13.3). Their most important functions are:

- Forms and maintains skin and body linings.
- Cements substances to promote strength in cells and hasten healing of injuries.
- Functions in all visual processes.
- Aids in the use of iron.

Sources of Vitamin A Remembering two simple colors —orange and green — will help you remember that foods of these colors will provide Vitamin A. Dark green, leafy, and orange vegetables (such as carrots, sweet potatoes, and greens) should be eaten regularly. Because Vitamin A is stored in the fat tissue of the body, an overdose through supplementation in pill form can be fatal. (The same is true for the other fat-soluble vitamins — D, E, and K.)

Sources of Vitamin C Vegetables such as broccoli, bell peppers, and spinach are recommended daily for supplying the needed catalyst Vitamin C. This vitamin is water-soluble, which means that if too much is taken in, the excess is excreted through the urine. If you decide to take Vitamin C supplement pills in massive doses, your body will react by increasing the level it needs. If you then stop taking Vitamin C supplements suddenly, your body will react as if it were deficient! Supplementation is costly and unnecessary for well people who eat properly.

FRUIT GROUP

Key ingredients are *folic acid, Vitamins A and C*, and fiber (Table 13.4).

TABLE 13.3   Ratings for Vegetable Group

Rating:	Food Choices in Ranked Order for Folic Acid and Vitamins A and C*
	red and green bell peppers bok choy spinach leaf lettuce broccoli carrots cauliflower
	cabbage, chard asparagus, kale vegetable juice, brussels sprouts iceberg lettuce, sweet potato tomato, snow peas zucchini, okra winter squash, green beans
	beets, cucumber celery, jicama artichoke, peas mushrooms
	eggplant, corn avocado, potato

*Based on 100-calorie portions.

TABLE 13.4   Ratings for Fruit Group

Rating:	Food Choices in Ranked Order for Folic Acid, Vitamins A and C
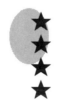	papaya strawberries kiwi orange, grapefruit orange juice cantaloupe mandarin oranges mango
	honeydew (melon) raspberries apricots rhubarb pineapple watermelon pineapple juice blueberries
	peach banana plum cherries frozen fruit juice bar canned fruit
	pears apples dried fruit grapes raisins

BREADS AND CEREALS GROUP

Although this group assists with the growth and maintenance of cells and with the elimination process (fiber provides bulk to your waste for easy removal), the major function is to provide *energy*. Your number-one daily need is energy to perform every daily function from sleeping to aerobics.

If you do not use this carbohydrate food for the expenditure of energy, for growth and repair, or eliminate it, you wear it as body fat — future energy. It's like constantly carrying around extra gasoline for your car. If you are an active person, such as a varsity or endurance athlete, you will want to provide an abundance of this energy food.

Key ingredients are *fiber, complex carbohydrates,* thiamine, iron, and niacin (Table 13.5).

TABLE 13.5	Ratings for Breads and Cereals Group
Rating:	**Food Choices in Ranked Order for Fiber and Complex Carbohydrates**

barley
bulgur
bran or whole-grain cereals
popcorn (air-popped or lite microwave)
whole-grain breads
oatmeal
whole-grain pasta
corn or whole-wheat tortilla

brown rice
bran muffin
whole-grain crackers
soft pretzel or breadstick
English muffin
enriched pasta
popcorn (oil-popped)

flour tortilla, bagel
enriched breads, enriched rice
pancakes, waffles
graham crackers, saltines
sweetened cereal
dry pretzels or breadsticks

cornbread
fruit or nut bread
biscuit, stuffing
croissant

SOMETIMES FOODS

The foods classified as extras have no recommended number of servings. These food choices provide little nutrition and often are high in sugar, salt, fat, and calories. Classified as extras are:

alcoholic beverages, bacon, bouillon, butter, cakes, candy, coffee, cookies, condiments, snack crackers, cream, regular fat cream cheese, doughnuts, french fries, fruit-flavored drinks, gelatin dessert, gravy, honey, jam, jelly, margarine, mayonnaise, nondairy creamer, olives, onion rings, pickles, pies, potato chips, salad dressings, sauces, seasonings, sherbet, soft drinks, sour cream, sugar, tea, tortilla chips, vegetable oils.[8]

SERVINGS PER DAY?[9]

The ranges given in Figure 13.3 are guides for how much food to eat each day. *Choose the lower or higher number of servings based on your calorie needs.* If you eat more or less than one serving, count as partial servings. For children under age 5, a serving is ¼–½ of a standard serving. However, to get enough calcium, all children need a total of at least 2 standard servings of milk or milk products each day.

The number of servings you need depends on how many calories you need, which in turn depends on your age, sex, physical condition, and how active you are. Almost everyone should have at least the minimum number of servings from each of the five major food groups daily. Many women, older children, and most teenagers and men need more. The top of the range is about right for an active man or a teenage boy.

To apply the guidelines on servings to your specific needs, Table 13.6 provides "Sample Diets for a Day at Three Calorie Levels."[10]

Monitoring Food/Beverage Intake

Do you eat a wide variety of foods in moderation as shown in the Food Guide Pyramid and as described in detail from the "Pyramid Plus" food groups? Begin to formulate your eating plan (Figure 13.4). Start by thinking about what you consumed today, and record the foods and beverages you ate and drank. Identify:

- nutrient density star rating (4/3/2/1/0);
- the appropriate food group for each item;
- the size/quantity of serving;
- with whom, where, why;
- duration of time taken to eat;
- other activity engaged in while eating;
- Chapter 14 also will request another entry, regarding your felt senses.

FIGURE 13.3   How Many Servings Do You Need Each Day?[9]

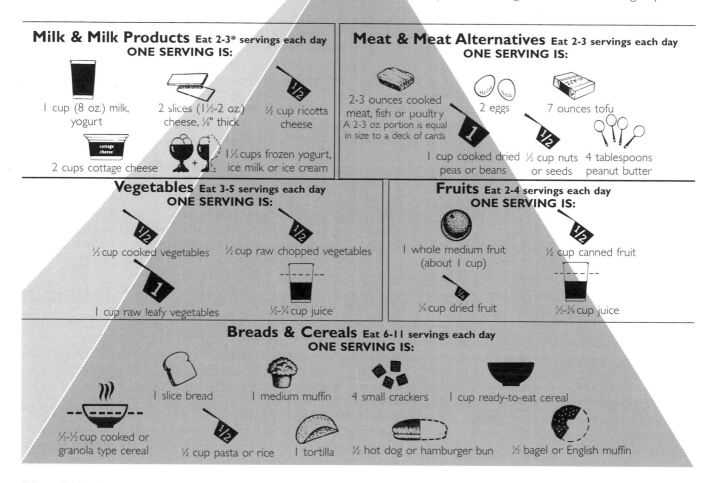

Sometimes Foods

Sometimes foods provide little or no nutrition and are often high in fat, sugar, salt and calories. They should be eaten in moderation and not in place of servings from the five food groups.

Milk & Milk Products Eat 2-3* servings each day
ONE SERVING IS:

I cup (8 oz.) milk, yogurt

2 slices (1½-2 oz.) cheese, ⅛" thick

½ cup ricotta cheese

2 cups cottage cheese

1½ cups frozen yogurt, ice milk or ice cream

Meat & Meat Alternatives Eat 2-3 servings each day
ONE SERVING IS:

2-3 ounces cooked meat, fish or poultry
A 2-3 oz. portion is equal in size to a deck of cards

2 eggs

7 ounces tofu

I cup cooked dried peas or beans

½ cup nuts or seeds

4 tablespoons peanut butter

Vegetables Eat 3-5 servings each day
ONE SERVING IS:

½ cup cooked vegetables

½ cup raw chopped vegetables

I cup raw leafy vegetables

½-¾ cup juice

Fruits Eat 2-4 servings each day
ONE SERVING IS:

I whole medium fruit (about I cup)

½ cup canned fruit

¼ cup dried fruit

½-¾ cup juice

Breads & Cereals Eat 6-11 servings each day
ONE SERVING IS:

I slice bread

I medium muffin

4 small crackers

I cup ready-to-eat cereal

⅓-½ cup cooked or granola type cereal

½ cup pasta or rice

I tortilla

½ hot dog or hamburger bun

½ bagel or English muffin

*Young Adults (11-24 years), Pregnant and Breastfeeding Women need 4 servings

Source: Nutrition Education Services / Oregon Dairy Council, "Pyramid Plus" pamphlet (Portland, OR: Oregon Dairy Council, 1994).

A "Food and Beverage Intake Diary for One Day" is provided in Chapter 15 (with space provided to record for one week).

For a combination food, think about what foods went into it and identify those foods with the appropriate food group. For example, the cheese on a pizza would be recorded in the Milk group, the tomatoes and any other vegetables in the Vegetable group, and the crust in the Breads group. The ingredients in a combination food may not always count as a full serving from the food group. Think in terms of quantity of servings, along with its nutrient category.

Continue monitoring your intake for one week. How does it measure up to the standards established for a balanced diet with special attention to selecting nutrient-dense foods? If your diet lacks variety, moderation, or foods from one of the food groups, you may not be getting all the nutrients and energy you need.

It's easy to improve your diet if you take it one step, one choice at a time. Start by choosing one challenge to work on, come up with a solution, and spend one week trying to correct it. After it's mastered, choose a second eating challenge, and then continue until you have a well-managed diet.

TABLE 13.6   Sample Diets for a Day at Three Calorie Levels[10]

	About 1,600	About 2,200	About 2,800
	1,600 calories is about right for many sedentary women and some older adults.	2,200 calories is about right for most children, teenage girls, active women, and many sedentary men. Women who are pregnant or breastfeeding may need somewhat more.	2,800 calories is about right for teenage boys, many active men, and some very active women.
Bread group servings	6	9	11
Fruit group servings	2	3	4
Vegetable group servings	3	4	5
Meat group	5 ounces	6 ounces	7 ounces
Milk group servings	2-3*	2-3*	2-3*
Total fat (grams)**	53	73	93
Total added sugars (teaspoons)**	6	12	18

*Women who are pregnant or breastfeeding, teenagers, and young adults to age 24 need 3 servings.

**See bulletin on fat and cholesterol for more information on how to count fat. See bulletin on sugar for more information on sugars[11]

Source: U.S. Department of Agriculture, Human Nutrition Information Service, Home and Garden Bulletin Number 253-2, p. 5, July 1993.

NUTRITION AND THE ATHLETE

The food groups already presented form the foundation of the diet recommended for young athletes. This plan serves as the nucleus for meals both in and out of athletic seasons. There is a vast leeway in the choice of foods within each of the food groups. Basic nutritional needs of athletes and nonathletes do not differ except in terms of calories.[12]

Total caloric needs vary with individual metabolism and physical activity. An intake of 2,000 calories each day should be the bare minimum allowed for an athlete involved in a vigorous training program. The number of calories a young male athlete expends in serious training may range as high as 4,000-6,000 calories per day. Calorie intake that exceeds expenditure for basal body functions, for physical activity, and for growth of lean body mass, however, will still form body fat, so pay attention to your training diet.

A pre-game meal should:

● Support blood sugar levels to avoid hunger sensations.
● Leave the stomach and upper bowel empty at the time of competition.
● Provide maximum hydration.
● Minimize stomach upset; promote maximum performance.
● Provide a psychological edge by including foods the athlete likes and believes will make him or her win.

FIGURE 13.4   Formulating an Eating Plan

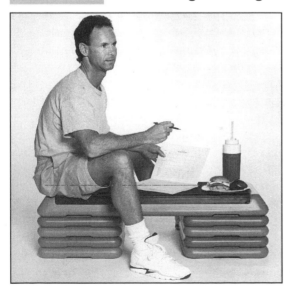

Carbohydrates in the diet will support blood sugar and provide glycogen stores to maintain these levels. Glycogen, the storage form of carbohydrate, seems to be the quickest and most efficient source of energy.

Good choices of high-carbohydrate foods are: apples, applesauce, bagels, baked potatoes, baking powder biscuits, bananas, boiled potatoes, bread (white, whole wheat), cheese pizza, egg noodles, graham crackers, hard rolls, macaroni and cheese, mashed potatoes, oatmeal, oranges and orange juice, orange sherbet, pancakes (enriched), pears, spaghetti, sponge cake, sweet potatoes, and waffles.

Carbohydrates are digested more rapidly than protein and fat. A breakfast of toast and jam, cereal with low-fat milk, and fruit or juice will leave the stomach much sooner than a meal of eggs with steak, sausage, or bacon.

Optimum hydration is important to athletes, especially those involved in endurance events, such as long-distance swimming and running. The immediate pre-game diet should consist of two to three glasses of some beverage, with no fewer than eight full glasses each 24 hours.

Whole milk is not recommended because of its high fat content. Caffeine also should be avoided because it may increase nervous tension and agitation before the contest. Noncarbonated fruit drinks are generally good choices.

Athletes should avoid concentrated sources of simple sugar such as glucose tablets and undiluted honey, as they can cause gas distention and discomfort. Also, bulky foods high in fiber or cellulose are not good choices before an event.

Athletes should avoid heavily salted foods on the day of competition, because these can cause water retention, which decreases athletic performance.

The pre-game meal should be eaten 3 to 4 hours before the contest. For a highly demanding sport, a 1,000-calorie meal is ideal. A 500-calorie meal suffices for a sport that requires lower energy.

Athletes must be prepared physically to meet the special demands on their bodies. The starting block is sound nutrition knowledge, and practice. If you sacrifice physical excellence to an inefficient or harmful diet, reduced strength and endurance and a poor performance will be the result.

Basic nutritional needs of athletes and nonathletes do not differ except in terms of calories.

DIETARY GUIDELINES FOR AMERICANS

Food alone cannot make a person healthy, but good eating habits based on moderation and variety can help keep a person healthy and even improve health. The following guidelines suggested for most Americans, developed by the U.S. Department of Agriculture, Human Nutrition Information Service, are printed in more detail in the eight-pamphlet series entitled, *Dietary Guidelines for Americans*.[13] In brief, most Americans need to pay more attention to the following guidelines.

● *Eat a variety of foods.* No single food supplies all the essential nutrients in the amounts you need. The greater the variety, the less likely you are to develop either a deficiency or an excess of any single nutrient.

● *Maintain healthy weight.* If you are too fat or too thin, your chances of developing health problems increase (for example, high blood pressure, diabetes, heart disease, certain cancers). There is no one plan for maintaining healthy weight. If your concern is to lose fat weight, increase your physical activity, eat slowly, eat less fat and fatty foods, eat less sugar and sweets, avoid too much alcohol, don't skip meals, and use up more calories than you take in. (Weight management is discussed in more detail in Chapter 14).

Choose a diet low in fat, and cholesterol. If you have a high blood cholesterol level, you have a greater chance of incurring a heart attack. A population such as that of the United States, with diets high in saturated fats and cholesterol, tend to produce high blood cholesterol levels.

Cholesterol is a necessary constituent of body tissues. When the circulating amount in the blood is higher than 200 milligrams (mg) (mild risk) or higher than 240 mg (high risk) it can cause early atherosclerosis. Atherosclerosis is a process of fatty build-up in the walls of the blood vessels, eventually leading to narrowing of the arteries and poor circulation. Cholesterol is one of the three major risk factors for coronary heart attack. (The other two are high blood pressure and cigarette smoking.)

High-density lipoproteins (HDL), also called "good cholesterol," coat the inside of the artery walls, providing a protective layer of grease to prevent fatty deposits from building up. They also serve as scavengers by actually *helping* dissolve fatty deposits when they do occur. A high amount in the blood indicates protection and decrease in heart attack risk. Certain people genetically have higher amounts. HDL also can be increased by weight loss and by regular aerobic exercise. A very low level in the blood indicates serious risk for heart attack.

Triglycerides (another type of fat) are diet-related and usually are not involved in the atherosclerosis process. High values occur in certain fat metabolism disorders and in diabetes.

Low-density lipoproteins (LDL) are responsive to dietary habits and form dangerous deposits on the walls of blood vessels, are the primary culprits in clogged arteries and atherosclerosis, and place a person at high risk for heart attack. If cholesterol and HDL values are borderline, LDL values may decide the risk.

Risk ratio is a calculated value (total cholesterol divided by your HDL value) that most experts use to predict an individual's risk of heart attack in coming years. Having a high HDL cholesterol value and low LDL cholesterol value reduces the risk.

Cholesterol is measured by a simple blood test that shows milligrams (mg) of total cholesterol (HDL, LDL, and VLDL) per deciliter (dl) of blood.

If your blood lipid values are high (see Table 13.7) and indicate increased risk for heart disease, you may benefit from improving your diet, increasing your exercise, or counseling concerning both.

There is controversy surrounding recommendations for healthy Americans. For the U.S. population as a whole, however, reducing the intake of total fat, saturated fat, and cholesterol is sensible.

● Choose lean meats, fish, poultry, dry beans, and peas as your protein sources.

● Moderate your intake of eggs and organ meats (such as liver).

● Limit your intake of butter, cream, hydrogenated margarines, shortenings, coconut oil, and foods made from those products.

● Trim excess fat from meats.

● Broil, bake, and boil rather than fry.

● Read food labels carefully to determine amounts and types of fat and cholesterol in foods.

● *Consume 300 mg/day or less of cholesterol.*

● Limit fat to 30% or less of total daily calories. To determine the percentage of calories in a product that come from fat: 1 gram of fat equals 9 calories. Multiply the grams of fat in a serving times 9. The result equals the number of calories from fat in a serving. Divide the fat calories by the total calories in a serving to determine the percent.

For example, if a chili label reads 1 cup serving = 200 calories/ fat, 10 g/ carbohydrate, 5 g/ sodium, 980 mg/: 1 cup of chili has 10 grams of fat.

$$10 \text{ g fat} \times 9 \text{ calories} = 90 \text{ calories from fat}$$
$$\text{in 1 cup}$$
$$90 \div 200 = 45\% \text{ of the calories in 1 cup of}$$
$$\text{chili come from fat.}[14]$$

● *Choose a diet with plenty of vegetables, fruits, and grain products.* The major sources of energy in the average U.S. diet are carbohydrates and fats. Carbohydrates have an advantage over fats: They contain less than half the number of calories per ounce than fats.

Complex carbohydrate foods are better than simple carbohydrates. Simple carbohydrates (sugars) provide calories for energy but little else in the way of nutrients. Complex carbohydrates (beans, nuts, fruits, whole-grain breads) contain many essential nutrients plus calories for energy.

Increasing your consumption of certain complex carbohydrates also can increase dietary fiber, which tends to reduce the symptoms of chronic constipation, diverticulosis, and some types of irritable bowel. Diets low in fiber content also might increase the risk of developing cancer of the colon. Eating fruits, vegetables, and whole-grain breads and cereals will provide adequate fiber in the diet. Goal-set to increase dietary fiber to 20-30 grams per day.

● *Use sugars in moderation.* The major hazard from eating too much sugar is tooth decay. The risk increases the more frequently you eat sugar and sweets, especially between meals, if you eat foods

TABLE 13.7	Blood Lipid Profile
Type	**Ideal**
Total cholesterol	<200 mg/deciliter (dl) of blood
High-density lipoprotein (HDL)	>50 mg/dl
Low-density lipoprotein (LDL)	<130 mg/dl
Triglycerides	35-180 mg/dl
Risk ratio = Your Total cholesterol ÷ HDL	Men <5:1 Women <4:1

that stick to the teeth (sticky candy, dates), and if you consume soft drinks throughout the day.

- Use less of all sugars (white, brown, raw, honey, and syrups).
- Select fresh fruit or fruit canned without heavy syrup.
- Read food labels for sugar information: If sucrose, glucose, maltose, dextrose, lactose, fructose, or syrup is listed as one of the first ingredients, the product has a lot of sugar.

To determine how many teaspoons of sugar a product contains: 5 grams of sugar equal 1 teaspoon.

Divide the grams in a serving by 5.
For example, if a cereal box label reads 1-cup
    serving = 140 calories/carbohydrates/starch,
    10 g/sucrose, 15 g/fiber 1 gm:
1 cup of cereal contains 15 grams.
15 grams of sucrose ÷ 5 = 3 teaspoons of simple
    sugar in 1 cup of cereal.

Products are healthier when sucrose (simple sugar) amounts are low.[15]

● *Use salt and sodium only in moderation.* The major hazard posed by excessive sodium is its effect on blood pressure. In populations where high-sodium intake is common, high blood pressure is also common. In populations with low-sodium intake, high blood pressure is rare. Establish preventive measures, such as:

- Eliminate all salt use at the table.
- Cook with little or no salt.
- Select foods that are low in sodium content.

The dietary goal for sodium intake is approximately 2,400 mg/day. The items in Table 13.8 have a relatively high sodium content.

● *If you drink alcoholic beverages, do so in moderation.* Alcoholic beverages tend to be high in calories and low in other nutrients. Heavy drinkers may lose their appetite for foods that contain essential nutrients. Vitamin and mineral deficiencies occur commonly in heavy drinkers because of poor nutrient intake and because alcohol alters absorption and use of some essential nutrients.

One or two drinks daily seem to cause no harm in adults, but even moderate drinkers should remember that alcohol is a high-calorie, low-nutrient food. If you wish to achieve or maintain ideal weight, alcohol intake must be well monitored. Women should consume no more than one drink a day, and men, no more than two drinks a day.

Recent research indicates that women have higher blood alcohol levels than men after having one drink. This is because women have less activity of an enzyme that helps metabolize alcohol in the body. Thus, women are more vulnerable to the acute and chronic complications of alcoholism.

Count a drink as:

- 12 fluid ounces of regular or light beer
- 5 fluid ounces of table wine
- 3½ fluid ounces of dessert wine
- 7 fluid ounces of light wine
- 1½ fluid ounces of gin, rum, whiskey (80 proof)
- 1 mixed drink[16]

THE NEW FOOD LABELS

The federal government has revamped the requirements on food labels significantly. The result is a label that is up-to-date with today's health concerns, a label you can understand, and one you can count on to help you plan healthy meals and snacks.

Front Label

What we eat actually can raise or lower our risks for acquiring certain diseases. For this reason, the Food and Drug Administration now is allowing claims linking a nutrient, or food, to the risk of a disease or health-related condition.[17] Only seven health messages are allowed because these are the only ones supported by scientific evidence. (e.g., "low fat") or ("a link between fruits and vegetables and a lower risk of cancer"). These claims must meet strict requirements enforced by the federal government, so when you see them, you can trust what they say. (Foods without the claims are not necessarily less nutritious.)

TABLE 13.8	**Relatively High Sodium-Content Foods**	
Food	Serving Size	Mg/Sodium Content
antacid (in water)	1 dose	564 mg.
canned corn	1 cup	384
cottage cheese	4 ounces	457
dill pickle	1	928
ham	3 ounces	1,114
salt	1 tsp.	1,938
tomato sauce	1 cup	1,498

Back/Side Label

The *side* or *back* of the package must feature a new nutrition panel (Figure 13.5). Almost all packaged foods will have to carry this nutrition information. Look for changes in *ingredient labeling* there, too. An ingredient list now is required on the labels of all foods with more than one ingredient.

NEW HEADING

The nutrition panel has a new title: "Nutrition Facts." It replaces "Nutrition Information Per Serving." When you see "Nutrition Facts," you know it's the correct food label.

FIGURE 13.5 Food Label

```
Nutrition Facts
Serving Size 1 cup (228g)
Servings Per Container 2

Amount Per Serving

Calories 250          Calories from Fat 110

                                   % Daily Value*

Total Fat 12g                              18%
    Saturated Fat 3g                       15%
Cholesterol 30mg                           10%
Sodium 470mg                               20%
Total Carbohydrate 31g                     10%
    Dietary Fiber 0g                        0%
    Sugars 5g
Protein 5g

Vitamin A      4%       •    Vitamin C     2%
Calcium       20%       •    Iron          4%

*Percent Daily Values are based on a 2,000 calorie
diet. Your daily values may be higher or lower
depending on your calorie needs:
```

		Calories	2,000	2,500
Total Fat	Less than		65g	80g
Sat Fat	Less than		20g	25g
Cholesterol	Less than		300mg	300mg
Sodium	Less than		2,400mg	2,400mg
Total Carbohydrate			300g	375g
Dietary Fiber			25g	30g

```
Calories per gram:
Fat 9   •   Carbohydrate 4   •   Protein 4
```

INGREDIENTS: WATER, ENRICHED MACARONI (ENRICHED FLOUR [NIACIN, FERROUS SULFATE (IRON), THIAMINE MONONITRATE AND RIBOFLAVIN], EGG WHITE), FLOUR, CHEDDAR CHEESE (MILK, CHEESE CULTURE, SALT, ENZYME), SPICES, MARGARINE (PARTIALLY HYDROGENATED SOYBEAN OIL, WATER, SOY LECITHIN, MONO- AND DIGLYCERIDES, BETA CAROTENE FOR COLOR, VITAMIN A PALMITATE), AND MALTODEXTRIN.

SERVING SIZES

The *serving size* is the basis for measuring a food's nutrient content and is the place to begin using Nutrition Facts. The new serving sizes are closer to amounts people really eat. If you choose to eat more, or less, than the serving size given on the label, adjust the amounts of nutrients accordingly.

NUTRIENT LISTING

Gone are the vitamins thiamine, riboflavin, and niacin (unless the label claims these or voluntarily lists them), because deficiencies of these no longer are a major problem in the United States. New listings include saturated fat, cholesterol, dietary fiber, and sugars. All other components of the former labeling system (such as sodium and iron) are still required.

% DAILY VALUES: THE KEY TO HEALTHY EATING

The amount of certain nutrients in a food now is expressed in two ways:

1. Amount by weight per serving.
2. As a percentage of the Daily Value (a unique nutritional reference tool).

By using the % Daily Values, you can determine easily whether a given food contributes a lot or a little of a specific nutrient. You also can compare different foods, with no need to do any calculations. A high percentage means the food contains a lot of a nutrient; a low percentage means it contains little. The goal is to choose a variety of foods that, together, give you close to 100% of each nutrient for a day, or average about 100% a day over several days.

The % Daily Values listed on the nutrition panel are based on consuming 2,000 calories a day. If you eat more or less, you'll need to adjust the values accordingly.

A CAVEAT

If you know little about human physiology — how your vital processes work — it's best not to resort to chance or whatever nutritional guidelines you encounter. An abundance of scientifically based, easy-to-read literature explains how to balance the needed nutrients. Select guidelines developed by well-established medical and fitness sources, such as those referred to in this chapter, rather than those from your favorite movie and television stars or supermarket trade magazines.

Goal Setting Challenge

You can set many possible small goals regarding nutrition. Begin by reviewing the chapter subtitles and listing topics or points that require your attention. Prioritize this list in order of need. Enjoy the challenge of balancing your intake (eating) with your expenditure (exercise). Or, if a course-goal is to lose fat weight or gain lean weight, *imbalancing* might be your goal.

Developing Goal Scripts for Chapter 13

DIRECTIONS: Write complete sentences for each segment below. Combine your responses to all four segments. This goal script is designed around your needs and choices. Read it (or make an audiotape and play it) twice daily, morning and evening, until you master it.

1 State one goal in positive, *present-tense* language. Ask yourself, "What will I experience — see, hear, taste, smell, feel — in regard to the results? Keep in mind that all powerful goals use the SMART formula: specific, measurable, achievable, realistic, timely.

_____

_____

2 State your *pleasure-value reasons.* Ask yourself, "Why am I totally committed to achieving this goal? What am I choosing to feel?"

_____

_____

3 State your *pain-avoidance value reasons.* Ask yourself, "What painful values do I choose to avoid feeling?"

_____

_____

4 State *immediate action(s)* you can take in the next 24 hours. Use positive, present-tense verbs such as *choose* and verbs ending with "ing."

_____

_____

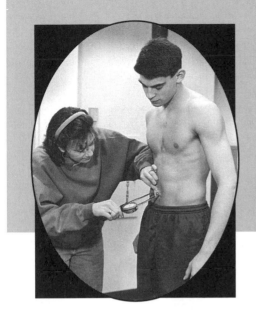

Weight Management

14

Your body is composed of two types of weight: lean weight and fat weight, also called lean body mass (or fat-free mass), and fat mass. Lean weight is composed primarily of bones, muscles, internal organs, and body fluids. It begins to weigh less after maturity when you stop growing at a certain steady pace every year. Fat weight is stored energy and protection for present and future use. The amount of each type of weight you carry is important to know so you can understand what is best for the health of your heart and lungs (cardiorespiratory system).

BODY FAT/BODY LEAN

Body fat can be classified as either essential fat or storage fat. *Essential fat* is needed for normal physiological functions. Without it, your health begins to deteriorate. This essential fat constitutes about 3% of the total fat in men and 10%–12% in women. The percentage is higher in women because it includes gender-related fat such as that found in the breast tissue, the uterus, and other gender-related areas.

Storage fat is the fat stored in adipose tissue, mostly beneath the skin (subcutaneous fat) and around major organs in the body. This fat serves three basic functions:

1. As an insulator to retain body heat;

2. As energy substrate for metabolism;

3. As padding against physical trauma to the body.

The amount of storage fat does not differ between men and women except that men tend to store fat around the waist and women more so around the hips and thighs.[1]

Each person can "wear" a certain percentage of fat to maintain ideal cardiorespiratory efficiency and minimize the risk factors associated with heart disease. Perhaps you are wearing less than a suggested ideal percentage of fat than is listed. This doesn't matter unless you are malnourishing yourself or you wish to look heavier cosmetically. A number of people don't wear ideal percentages. For example, endurance athletes such as marathon runners and Olympic gymnasts carry much less fat. They burn it off and don't carry the excess. They usually eat right to provide the necessary nutrients and energy and thus display a firm, trim, toned look, yet they stay well.

In contrast are individuals who have the "starvation disease" anorexia nervosa. They, too, carry less than the suggested ideal percentage of body fat, but they do this by also eliminating their lean weight. They desire a trim look but go about it in a way that is against all physiological principles of proper weight loss. To them, weight loss means dropping pounds to be slim at all cost, no matter what kind of weight it is, fat or lean. This is an extremely detrimental way to lose weight. The concept of healthy slimness and unhealthy slimness is presented later in the chapter.

DETERMINING YOUR BODY COMPOSITION

Ideal weight cannot be determined just by looking at someone. An assessment of body composition involves determining as precisely as possible an individual's body fat and lean body weight. This enables an accurate estimate of ideal weight. The traditional standardized weight tables, adjusted for gender, height and frame size, have been shown to be grossly inaccurate for many people. The ideal weight within any one category of these tables can vary up to 22 pounds. Individuals often fall within the normal range for their category but actually can have 10 to 30 pounds of excess body fat.

Measurement techniques now can determine more accurately whether an individual is overweight (overfat) or obese, and quantify exactly by how much.

Because of the ease of use in a fitness class setting and the availability of equipment, the skinfold thickness technique is used most often with this population. Body composition is assessed to determine lean weight mass and percentage of body fat. With that information, an estimated ideal body weight can be established that is best for your cardiorespiratory health.

Measuring Skinfold Thickness

Assessment of body composition using skinfold thickness is based on the principle that approximately half of the body's fatty tissue is deposited directly beneath the skin. If this tissue is estimated validly and reliably, it can produce a good indication of percent body fat.

This test is done with the aid of a precision instrument called a *skinfold caliper*. Three specific sites must be measured with the calipers and then added together to reflect the total percentage of fat. These measurements may vary slightly on the same subject when they are taken by different professionals. Therefore, pre- and post-measurements preferably should be taken by the same technician.

Using the three-site skinfold testing, the procedure for assessing percent body fat follows:

1. Specific anatomical sites are tested. For men, these are the chest, abdomen, and thigh (Figure 14.1). For women, the triceps, suprailium, and thigh areas are tested (Figure 14.2). All measurements should be taken on the right side of the

---

FIGURE 14.1

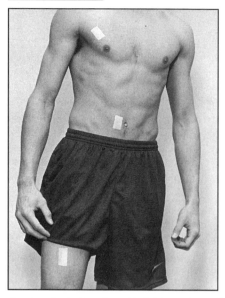

Anatomical sites for skinfold testing of men.

FIGURE 14.2

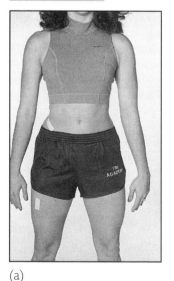 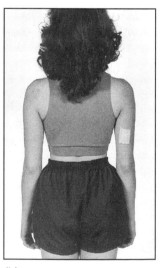

(a)   (b)

Anatomical sites for skinfold testing of women.

body with the subject standing. The correct anatomical landmarks for skinfolds are:

MEN

Chest: A diagonal fold halfway between the shoulder crease and the nipple.

Abdomen: A vertical fold taken about 1" to the right of the umbilicus.

Thigh: A vertical fold on the front of the right thigh, midway between the knee and hip. (Weight-bear on left foot.)

WOMEN

Suprailium: A diagonal fold above the crest of the ilium (on the side of the hip) (a).

Thigh: A vertical fold on the front of the right thigh, midway between the knee and hip (a). (Weight-bear on left foot.)

Triceps: A vertical fold on the back of the upper arm, halfway between the shoulder and the elbow (b).

2. The technician conducts the measurements by grasping a thickness of skin in the key locations just mentioned, with a thumb and forefinger, and pulling the fold slightly away from the muscular tissue. The calipers are held perpendicular to the fold, and the measurement is taken ½" below the finger hold. Each site is measured three times, and the values are read to the nearest .1 to .5 mm. The average of the two closest readings is recorded as your final value. The readings are taken in close succession to avoid excessive compression of the skinfold. Releasing and regrabbing the skinfold is required between readings.

3. When doing pre- and post-assessments, the measurement should be conducted at the same time of day. The best time is early in the morning to avoid hydration changes resulting from activity or exercise.

Determining Your Percent Body Fat

The percent fat is obtained by adding all three skinfold measurements and looking up the respective values on Table 14.1 for women, 14.2 for men under 40, and 14.3 for men over 40. Record your findings in Figure 14.3.

TABLE 14.1

Percent Fat Estimates for Women Calculated from Triceps, Suprailium, and Thigh Skinfold Thickness

Sum of 3 Skin-folds	Under 22	23 to 27	28 to 32	33 to 37	38 to 42	43 to 47	48 to 52	53 to 57	Over 58
23-25	9.7	9.9	10.2	10.4	10.7	10.9	11.2	11.4	11.7
26-28	11.0	11.2	11.5	11.7	12.0	12.3	12.5	12.7	13.0
29-31	12.3	12.5	12.8	13.0	13.3	13.5	13.8	14.0	14.3
32-34	13.6	13.8	14.0	14.3	14.5	14.8	15.0	15.3	15.5
35-37	14.8	15.0	15.3	15.5	15.8	16.0	16.3	16.5	16.8
38-40	16.0	16.3	16.5	16.7	17.0	17.2	17.5	17.7	18.0
41-43	17.2	17.4	17.7	17.9	18.2	18.4	18.7	18.9	19.2
44-46	18.3	18.6	18.8	19.1	19.3	19.6	19.8	20.1	20.3
47-49	19.5	19.7	20.0	20.2	20.5	20.7	21.0	21.2	21.5
50-52	20.6	20.8	21.1	21.3	21.6	21.8	22.1	22.3	22.6
53-55	21.7	21.9	22.1	22.4	22.6	22.9	23.1	23.4	23.6
56-58	22.7	23.0	23.2	23.4	23.7	23.9	24.2	24.4	24.7
59-61	23.7	24.0	24.2	24.5	24.7	25.0	25.2	25.5	25.7
62-64	24.7	25.0	25.2	25.5	25.7	26.0	26.2	26.4	26.7
65-67	25.7	25.9	26.2	26.4	26.7	26.9	27.2	27.4	27.7
68-70	26.6	26.9	27.1	27.4	27.6	27.9	28.1	28.4	28.6
71-73	27.5	27.8	28.0	28.3	28.5	28.8	29.0	29.3	29.5
74-76	28.4	28.7	28.9	29.2	29.4	29.7	29.9	30.2	30.4
77-79	29.3	29.5	29.8	30.0	30.3	30.5	30.8	31.0	31.3
80-82	30.1	30.4	30.6	30.9	31.1	31.4	31.6	31.9	32.1
83-85	30.9	31.2	31.4	31.7	31.9	32.2	32.4	32.7	32.9
86-88	31.7	32.0	32.2	32.5	32.7	32.9	33.2	33.4	33.7
89-91	32.5	32.7	33.0	33.2	33.5	33.7	33.9	34.2	34.4
92-94	33.2	33.4	33.7	33.9	34.2	34.4	34.7	34.9	35.2
95-97	33.9	34.1	34.4	34.6	34.9	35.1	35.4	35.6	35.9
98-100	34.6	34.8	35.1	35.3	35.5	35.8	36.0	36.3	36.5
101-103	35.2	35.4	35.7	35.9	36.2	36.4	36.7	36.9	37.2
104-106	35.8	36.1	36.3	36.6	36.8	37.1	37.3	37.5	37.8
107-109	36.4	36.7	36.9	37.1	37.4	37.6	37.9	38.1	38.4
110-112	37.0	37.2	37.5	37.7	38.0	38.2	38.5	38.7	38.9
113-115	37.5	37.8	38.0	38.2	38.5	38.7	39.0	39.2	39.5
116-118	38.0	38.3	38.5	38.8	39.0	39.3	39.5	39.7	40.0
119-121	38.5	38.7	39.0	39.2	39.5	39.7	40.0	40.2	40.5
122-124	39.0	39.2	39.4	39.7	39.9	40.2	40.4	40.7	40.9
125-127	39.4	39.6	39.9	40.1	40.4	40.6	40.9	41.1	41.4
128-130	39.8	40.0	40.3	40.5	40.8	41.0	41.3	41.5	41.8

NOTE: Body density is calculated based on the generalized equation for predicting body density of women developed by A. S. Jackson, M. L. Pollock, and A. Ward. *Medicine and Science in Sports and Exercise* 12:175-182, 1980. Percent body fat is determined from the calculated body density using the Siri formula.

TABLE 14.2

Percent Fat Estimates for Men Under 40 Calculated from Chest, Abdomen, and Thigh Skinfold Thickness

Sum of 3 Skin-folds	Under 19	20 to 22	23 to 25	26 to 28	29 to 31	32 to 34	35 to 37	38 to 40
					Age to the Last Year			
8-10	.9	1.3	1.6	2.0	2.3	2.7	3.0	3.3
11-13	1.9	2.3	2.6	3.0	3.3	3.7	4.0	4.3
14-16	2.9	3.3	3.6	3.9	4.3	4.6	5.0	5.3
17-19	3.9	4.2	4.6	4.9	5.3	5.6	6.0	6.3
20-22	4.8	5.2	5.5	5.9	6.2	6.6	6.9	7.3
23-25	5.8	6.2	6.5	6.8	7.2	7.5	7.9	8.2
26-28	6.8	7.1	7.5	7.8	8.1	8.5	8.8	9.2
29-31	7.7	8.0	8.4	8.7	9.1	9.4	9.8	10.1
32-34	8.6	9.0	9.3	9.7	10.0	10.4	10.7	11.1
35-37	9.5	9.9	10.2	10.6	10.9	11.3	11.6	12.0
38-40	10.5	10.8	11.2	11.5	11.8	12.2	12.5	12.9
41-43	11.4	11.7	12.1	12.4	12.7	13.1	13.4	13.8
44-46	12.2	12.6	12.9	13.3	13.6	14.0	14.3	14.7
47-49	13.1	13.5	13.8	14.2	14.5	14.9	15.2	15.5
50-52	14.0	14.3	14.7	15.0	15.4	15.7	16.1	16.4
53-55	14.8	15.2	15.5	15.9	16.2	16.6	16.9	17.3
56-58	15.7	16.0	16.4	16.7	17.1	17.4	17.8	18.1
59-61	16.5	16.9	17.2	17.6	17.9	18.3	18.6	19.0
62-64	17.4	17.7	18.1	18.4	18.8	19.1	19.4	19.8
65-67	18.2	18.5	18.9	19.2	19.6	19.9	20.3	20.6
68-70	19.0	19.3	19.7	20.0	20.4	20.7	21.1	21.4
71-73	19.8	20.1	20.5	20.8	21.2	21.5	21.9	22.2
74-76	20.6	20.9	21.3	21.6	22.0	22.2	22.7	23.0
77-79	21.4	21.7	22.1	22.4	22.8	23.1	23.4	23.8
80-82	22.1	22.5	22.8	23.2	23.5	23.9	24.2	24.6
83-85	22.9	23.2	23.6	23.9	24.3	24.6	25.0	25.3
86-88	23.6	24.0	24.3	24.7	25.0	25.4	25.7	26.1
89-91	24.4	24.7	25.1	25.4	25.8	26.1	26.5	26.8
92-94	25.1	25.5	25.8	26.2	26.5	26.9	27.2	27.5
95-97	25.8	26.2	26.5	26.9	27.2	27.6	27.9	28.3
98-100	26.6	26.9	27.3	27.6	27.9	28.3	28.6	29.0
101-103	27.3	27.6	28.0	28.3	28.6	29.0	29.3	29.7
104-106	27.9	28.3	28.6	29.0	29.3	29.7	30.0	30.4
107-109	28.6	29.0	29.3	29.7	30.0	30.4	30.7	31.1
110-112	29.3	29.6	30.0	30.3	30.7	31.0	31.4	31.7
113-115	30.0	30.3	30.7	31.0	31.3	31.7	32.0	32.4
116-118	30.6	31.0	31.3	31.6	32.0	32.3	32.7	33.0
119-121	31.3	31.6	32.0	32.3	32.6	33.0	33.3	33.7
122-124	31.9	32.2	32.6	32.9	33.3	33.6	34.0	34.3
125-127	32.5	32.9	33.2	33.5	33.9	34.2	34.6	34.9
128-130	33.1	33.5	33.8	34.2	34.5	34.9	35.2	35.5

NOTE: Body density is calculated based on the generalized equation for predicting body density of men developed by A. S. Jackson, M. L. Pollock. *British Journal of Nutrition* 40:497-504, 1978. Percent body fat is determined from the calculated body density using the Siri formula.

TABLE 14.3

Percent Fat Estimates for Men Over 40 Calculated from Chest, Abdomen, and Thigh Skinfold Thickness

Sum of 3 Skin-folds	41 to 43	44 to 46	47 to 49	50 to 52	53 to 55	56 to 58	59 to 61	Over 62
					Age to the Last Year			
8-10	3.7	4.0	4.4	4.7	5.1	5.4	5.8	6.1
11-13	4.7	5.0	5.4	5.7	6.1	6.4	6.8	7.1
14-16	5.7	6.0	6.4	6.7	7.1	7.4	7.8	8.1
17-19	6.7	7.0	7.4	7.7	8.1	8.4	8.7	9.1
20-22	7.6	8.0	8.3	8.7	9.0	9.4	9.7	10.1
23-25	8.6	8.9	9.3	9.6	10.0	10.3	10.7	11.0
26-28	9.5	9.9	10.2	10.6	10.9	11.3	11.6	12.0
29-31	10.5	10.8	11.2	11.5	11.9	12.2	12.6	12.9
32-34	11.4	11.8	12.1	12.4	12.8	13.1	13.5	13.8
35-37	12.3	12.7	13.0	13.4	13.7	14.1	14.4	14.8
38-40	13.2	13.6	13.9	14.3	14.6	15.0	15.3	15.7
41-43	14.1	14.5	14.8	15.2	15.5	15.9	16.2	16.6
44-46	15.0	15.4	15.7	16.1	16.4	16.8	17.1	17.5
47-49	15.9	16.2	16.6	16.9	17.3	17.6	18.0	18.3
50-52	16.8	17.1	17.5	17.8	18.2	18.5	18.8	19.2
53-55	17.6	18.0	18.3	18.7	19.0	19.4	19.7	20.1
56-58	18.5	18.8	19.2	19.5	19.9	20.2	20.6	20.9
59-61	19.3	19.7	20.0	20.4	20.7	21.0	21.4	21.7
62-64	20.1	20.5	20.8	21.2	21.5	21.9	22.2	22.6
65-67	21.0	21.3	21.7	22.0	22.4	22.7	23.0	23.4
68-70	21.8	22.1	22.5	22.8	23.2	23.5	23.9	24.2
71-73	22.6	22.9	23.3	23.6	24.0	24.3	24.7	25.0
74-76	23.4	23.7	24.1	24.4	24.8	25.1	25.4	25.8
77-79	24.1	24.5	24.8	25.2	25.5	25.9	26.2	26.6
80-82	24.9	25.3	25.6	26.0	26.3	26.6	27.0	27.3
83-85	25.7	26.0	26.4	26.7	27.1	27.4	27.8	28.1
86-88	26.4	26.8	27.1	27.5	27.8	28.2	28.5	28.9
89-91	27.2	27.5	27.9	28.2	28.6	28.9	29.2	29.6
92-94	27.9	28.2	28.6	28.9	29.3	29.6	30.0	30.3
95-97	28.6	29.0	29.3	29.7	30.0	30.4	30.7	31.1
98-100	29.3	29.7	30.0	30.4	30.7	31.1	31.4	31.8
101-103	30.0	30.4	30.7	31.1	31.4	31.8	32.1	32.5
104-106	30.7	31.1	31.4	31.8	32.1	32.5	32.8	33.2
107-109	31.4	31.8	32.1	32.4	32.8	33.1	33.5	33.8
110-112	32.1	32.4	32.8	33.1	33.5	33.8	34.2	34.5
113-115	32.7	33.1	33.4	33.8	34.1	34.5	34.8	35.2
116-118	33.4	33.7	34.1	34.4	34.8	35.1	35.5	35.8
119-121	34.0	34.4	34.7	35.1	35.4	35.8	36.1	36.5
122-124	34.7	35.0	35.4	35.7	36.1	36.4	36.7	37.1
125-127	35.3	35.6	36.0	36.3	36.7	37.0	37.4	37.7
128-130	35.9	36.2	36.6	36.9	37.3	37.6	38.0	38.5

NOTE: Body density is calculated based on the generalized equation for predicting body density of men developed by A. S. Jackson, M. L. Pollock. *British Journal of Nutrition* 40:497-504, 1978. Percent body fat is determined from the calculated body density using the Siri formula.

FIGURE 14.3   Calculating Your Percent Body Fat

Record your three skinfold readings, add them together, and record total value.

_____

_____

_____

_____ Total of 3 skinfold readings

Using Tables 14.1, 14.2, or 14.3, determine your current percent body fat according to your age and gender and record it here:

_____ • _____ **%**

My current classification label is:_____.

Determining Your Classification

After finding out your percent body fat, you can determine your current body composition classification according to Table 14.4. In this table you will find the "health fitness" and the "high physical fitness" percent fat standards. For example, the recommended health fitness fat percentage for a 20-year-old female is 28% or less. The health fitness standard is established at the point where there seems to be no detriment to health in terms of percent body fat. A high physical fitness range for this same woman is between 18% and 23%.

The high physical fitness standard does not mean that you cannot be somewhat below this number. As mentioned earlier, many highly trained athletes measurements are below the percentages set. _The 3% essential fat for men and 12% for women are the lower limits for people to maintain good health._ Below these percentages, normal physiologic functions can be seriously impaired.

TABLE 14.4

Body Composition Classification According to Percent Body Fat

MEN

Age	Excellent	Good	Moderate	Overweight	Obese
≤19	12.0	12.1-17.0	17.1-22.0	22.1-27.0	≥27.1
20-29	13.0	13.1-18.0	18.1-23.0	23.1-28.0	≥28.1
30-39	14.0	14.1-19.0	19.1-24.0	24.1-29.0	≥29.1
40-49	15.0	15.1-20.0	20.1-25.0	25.1-30.0	≥30.1
≥50	16.0	16.1-21.5	21.1-26.0	26.1-31.0	≥31.1

WOMEN

Age	Excellent	Good	Moderate	Overweight	Obese
≤19	17.0	17.1-22.0	22.1-27.0	27.1-32.0	≥32.1
20-29	18.0	18.1-23.0	23.1-28.0	28.1-33.0	≥33.1
30-39	19.0	19.1-24.0	24.1-29.0	29.1-34.0	≥34.1
40-49	20.0	20.1-25.0	25.1-30.0	30.1-35.0	≥35.1
≥50	21.0	21.1-26.5	26.1-31.0	31.1-36.0	≥36.1

▣ "High physical fitness" standard

▣ "Health fitness" standard

Source: From _Principles & Labs for Physical Fitness & Wellness_ by Werner W. K. Hoeger (Englewood, CO: Morton Publishing Company, 1994), p. 62.

In addition, some experts point out that a little storage fat (over the essential fat) is better than none at all. As a result, the health and high fitness standards for percent fat in Table 14.4 are set higher than the minimum essential fat requirements, at a point conducive to optimal health and well-being. Also, because lean tissue decreases with age, one extra percentage point is allowed for every additional decade of life.

ACHIEVING A HEALTHY SLIMNESS

We seem to admit readily that a primary goal in taking fitness courses is to *appear* healthy and slim. We desire this goal because we can see directly when our body looks nice, lean, and toned; likewise, we can see directly when it looks out of shape and flabby. Many individuals therefore focus initially on a form of "fitness" or "being in shape" that they can readily see.

Your outer appearance, however, is not the entire, or even major, focus of a quality fitness program. You can live without well-toned muscles or a trim figure, but you can't live very long without a strong heart and lungs. Looking attractive and feeling good about your appearance are good ancillary goals (Figure 14.4). The key word, however, is *healthy* slimness. This will require developing a weight management program. To calculate your recommended body weight see Figure 14.5.

FIGURE 14.4

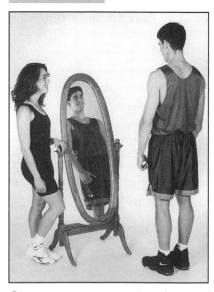

Outer appearance, a secondary goal.

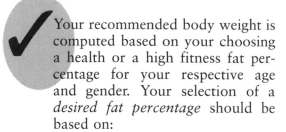

Goal Setting Challenge

Your recommended body weight is computed based on your choosing a health or a high fitness fat percentage for your respective age and gender. Your selection of a *desired fat percentage* should be based on:

● your current percent body fat; and

● your personal health-fitness goals and objectives.

Select your desired/recommended body fat percentage from Table 14.4 based on your goals and the "health" or "high fitness" standards given. Express this percentage in decimal form:

._____% (RFP) GOAL

TIMEFRAME: _____

PRINCIPLES OF WEIGHT MANAGEMENT

Weight management means controlling the amount of body fat in relation to the amount of lean tissue. Principles of weight management include:

1. *Weight maintenance* (keeping the same ratio of fat to amount of lean you're currently carrying).

2. *Weight gain* (almost always in terms of lean weight gain, not fat weight gain).

3. *Weight loss* (always in terms of loss of body fat).

Weight Maintenance

In regard to weight maintenance:

● Your current composition of fat to lean is ideal for your best cardiorespiratory health.

● You are pleased with how you look. You have enough strength to function well in your daily life of work and recreation, to whatever extreme that may encompass. To remain at this constant weight, your energy must be in balance:

calories in (eating) = calories out (exercise).

FIGURE 14.5

DETERMINING YOUR RECOMMENDED BODY WEIGHT

1. **Fat Weight:** Multyply your total body weight in pounds (BW) by the current percent fat (%F) you're carrying (see Tables 14.1, 14.2, and 14.3), expressing this percentage in decimal form. (BW × ._____ %F). This is your *fat weight* (FW), the actual number of pounds of fat you now carry.

2. **Lean Weight:** Subtract your fat weight (FW) from your total body weight (BW − FW). This is your current *lean weight* (LW).

3. Place your desired/**recommended *fat percentage*** (RFP) you selected here (see Goal Setting Challenge on previous page), expressing this percentage in decimal form:

4. **Recommended or Ideal Weight:** To calculate your recommended or ideal weight, use the following formula: LW ÷ (1.0 − .RFP) = RW (Recommended or Ideal Weight).

GOAL: Subtract your recommended body weight from your current weight (BW − RW). This tells you exactly how many pounds you'll goal-set to lose or gain. (Positive numbers = Weight to *lose*. Negative numbers = weight to *gain*.)

CALCULATE HERE:

_____ × ._____ = _____
(BW   ×   % F   =   FW)

_____ − _____ = _____
(BW   −   FW   =   LW)

._____ % (RFP)

_____ ÷ (1.0 − .____) = ____
LW   RFP   RW

_____ − RW = _____
BW   Actual pounds
                   I'm Goal Setting to
                   lose/gain.

Example: A 19-year-old-female who weighs 136 pounds and is 25% fat would like to know what her recommended or ideal weight should be, with a "desired"/recommended fat percentage of 17%, which is the "high physical fitness" standard.

Sex: female
Age: 19
BW: 136 lbs
%F: 25% (.25 in decimal form)
RFP: 17% (.17 in decimal form)

- FW = BW × %F
  FW = 136 × .25 = 34 lbs.
- LW = BW − FW
  LW = 136 − 34 = 102 lbs.
- RFP: 17% (.17 in decimal form)
- RW = LW ÷ (1.0 − .RFP)
  RW = 102 ÷ (1.0 − .17)
  RW = 102 ÷ (.83) = 122.9 lbs.*

*(Recommended Body Weight)

GOAL: To reach her recommended/ideal body weight, she'll choose to goal-set to lose 13.1 pounds of fat weight (subtracting *recommended body weight from the weight she is currently at (136 − 122.9 = 13.1).

TIMEFRAME:

_____ /
              1 wk

_____ /
              1 mo

_____ /
              3 mo

_____ /
              6 mo

_____ /
              1 yr

Because "calories out" declines with aging (your metabolism slows down and you are less active), a decline in "calories in" (eating less) must accompany the aging processes.

Weight Gain

Weight gain almost always refers to gaining *lean* tissue, or thickening muscle fiber. When you want to look better cosmetically or to increase your strength for a sport or for daily needs, weight training is the type of activity in which to engage. If you are at an overfat weight, to *gain lean weight and lose extra body fat* simultaneously will require you to eat less while providing the *increased exercise* of weight training. Only if you are at ideal weight or underfat weight should you accompany this weight-gain program with an increase in caloric intake.[2]

Weight gain, then, means increasing muscle mass, or thickening of muscle fibers. You do not gain more muscle cells; you thicken what you presently have.

Weight Loss

Weight loss refers to purposefully losing *fat weight*, never lean weight. Weight loss, of course, can be both lean and fat, according to how you go about losing the weight. Before you spend your money on any unique new weight reduction plan, claim, product, device, or book, call your local Better Business Bureau. If you completely understand the principles of weight loss, you will be able to determine a product's or program's worth before you spend time, money, and energy on it. These principles are as follows.

1. *Fat weight is the only kind of weight to lose.* If a product or program claims to "get rid of excess body fluids," beware! Body fluids are not fat. Unnatural water retention, *edema*, is a condition to be monitored and treated by a doctor, not by self-prescribed procedures or products.

2. *If water weight (fluid) is lost by sweating during exercise, it will and should return in 24 hours* to maintain the body's synchronized chemical balance. The energy-producing (metabolic) processes perform best when all of the necessary components are present. Dropping water weight is not effective weight loss. It is part of the fat-free weight and is vital to continuous well-being. You can understand, then, why weighing yourself

after a strenuous exercise session is an inaccurate time to weigh.

3. *Fat is metabolized more readily and efficiently by performing moderate-intensity exercise for a long time.* If you are able to work continuously at a moderate intensity (lower end of your training zone), for more than 30 minutes, you will tap into the most physiologically sound way to metabolize (burn off) unwanted body fat. You need to exercise for *more than 30 minutes at a time to make significant changes in the fat content of the body.*

   Wearing rubber suits, transparent plastic wrap around body parts, or heavy, long-sleeved sweats, pantyhose, or tights on hot days inhibits the free flow of sweat and does not allow it to perform its function of cooling. In hot and humid settings, wear as little as possible when performing fitness exercises. You cannot metabolize (burn up) fat faster by wearing more clothes.

4. *Fat burns off your body in a general way.* You can't "spot-reduce." Spot-reducing is perhaps the most prevalent misconception concerning fat weight loss. Many unscrupulous people are defrauding unsuspecting overfat Americans out of millions of dollars every year.

   By your genetic constitution, your body will use up its stored energy (fat) any way it is programmed to do. You cannot do fifty leg lifts a day and hope to reduce the fat deposits in the area. You will shape up (thicken) the muscle fiber in the area, and toned muscles contain more of the enzymes involved in breaking down fat, but you do not burn off the fat there or at any specific location. As energy is needed, it is withdrawn first from the immediate sources, and when this is used up, randomly from more permanent storage. It then is converted to an immediate usable form. Thus, at first you may lose weight in places you don't necessarily wish to, such as your face or chest/breast area. With perseverance, however, you'll burn off the fat in problem areas, too.

5. *Fat weight loss is accomplished most readily through a combined program of monitoring your food intake carefully and exercising aerobically.* When you monitor food intake (and eat less) and exercise (expend more calories or energy), you lose almost 100% fat. This is the only kind of weight you want to lose. Exercise speeds weight loss, not only by burning calories

while you're working out but also by revitalizing your metabolism so you continue to burn calories more readily for the next few hours.

Losing fat weight by simply eating less food is difficult. If you avoid exercise and choose to severely restrict food intake only, when you step on a scale the weight loss is not just fat. According to the way in which you have "dieted," your weight loss is approximately one-half to two-thirds fat loss and *one-third to one-half lean weight loss*. If your lifestyle and habits of eating and exercising don't change after you stop "dieting" and you gain back your lost weight, what you gain back is all fat. You are worse off because you lost both fat and lean and regained only fat. Over a lifetime of "yo-yo" crash dieting, the entire body composition is changing detrimentally.

You can *lose* fat weight in many ways. Research has determined that the only way to *keep* fat weight off is by following a regular exercise program.[3]

6. *Weight can be both gained and lost through an endurance exercise program.* You will be burning off fat for energy and building up muscle simultaneously. Therefore, if you do not see a change on the scale immediately, don't be disappointed.

7. *A light exercise program tends to increase appetite, and a strenuous exercise program decreases appetite.* After an endurance (aerobic) hour, the desire for food diminishes greatly. You will have time to carefully select or prepare what you know is good for you rather than ravenously grab that easy, high-calorie junk food just sitting around.

8. *Eating less food is easier than exercising it off.* In most high-intensity fitness sessions, you will burn only about 300 calories. If you are seriously interested in losing extra fat weight, think twice about rewarding yourself with high-caloric treats afterward. Instead, replenish your water loss with noncaloric, yet quite filling, ice water.

9. *There is no such thing as a constipated endurance aerobic exerciser or athlete.* Regular, rhythmic stimulation of the entire digestion and elimination processes is one of the side benefits of aerobic exercise.

10. *The body's energy balance determines whether a person gains or loses body fat.* Proper weight loss is simply the result of *taking in less caloric energy and expending more.*

WEIGHT-LOSS STRATEGIES

The challenge involved in being overweight may involve the need for any of the following: (a) a better self-image, (b) a naturally slender eating strategy, (c) learning effective ways to become motivated and make decisions, (d) resolving a phobic response to childhood abuse, (e) learning better social skills, or (f) learning better coping skills.[4]

"Naturally Slender" Eating

One of the main differences between naturally slender people and overweight individuals is the construction of their mental images and self-talk concerning food. Overweight people usually construct *present-tense* pictures and self-talk. They see, smell, hear, experience food, and state internally, "Boy, am I hungry!" The result is that they eat immediately. They focus only on the pleasurable taste of food as they eat.

Naturally thin people usually do not have this present-tense strategy. They create *future-tense* pictures, self-talk, and feelings. They experience how they'll feel over time[5] (see Figure 14.6). Naturally slender people, as they approach a restaurant food bar or order from a menu, determine *ahead of time* how they choose to feel *when they are all finished eating*. This proactive, plan-ahead approach can be the difference between being naturally slender or being overweight for a lifetime.

FIGURE 14.6

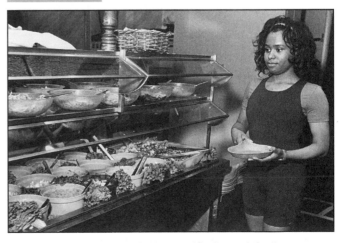

Creating future-tense pictures, self-talk, and feelings.

Control Panel With One Large Dial

The control panel was introduced in Chapter 12 to rate the tension and relaxation experienced from stressors. This same type of control panel can be used in an eating strategy, to reflect how "empty" or "full" you feel:

— before you eat;
— during the meal;
— when you're done eating.

Before you select, you have to "go inside" where your hunger cues are, and predetermine how empty or full you are. Give that feeling a number from 0 to 10 and an accompanying label, as shown in Figure 14.7.

Then, when selecting and eating food, imagine your control panel and adjust it to how you feel currently, how you choose to feel during the eating process, and how you choose to feel when you're done eating and drinking. Add this 'feeling sense' to the one-week monitoring of your eating and beverage intake forms found in Chapter 15.

Caloric Intake and Use

Everything you eat or drink becomes "you" for either a short or a long time. You are what you eat and drink. The food nutrients you eat maintain basic body functions such as breathing, blood circulation, normal body temperature, and growth and repair of all tissue. These are related to fixed factors such as age, body size, and physiological state. Any kind of caloric intake your body doesn't use or doesn't eliminate through solid or liquid waste is kept and worn as body fat for future energy needs.

FIGURE 14.7 Control Panel with One Large Dial

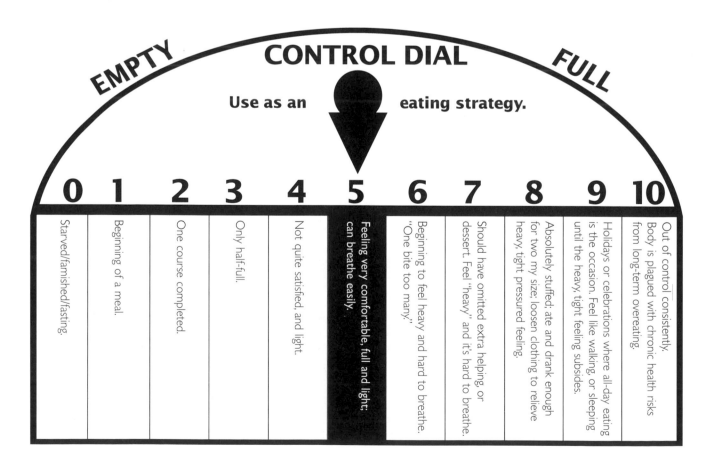

EMPTY CONTROL DIAL FULL

Use as an eating strategy.

0	1	2	3	4	5	6	7	8	9	10
Starved/famished/fasting.	Beginning of a meal.	One course completed.	Only half-full.	Not quite satisfied, and light.	Feeling very comfortable, full and light; can breathe easily.	Beginning to feel heavy and hard to breathe. "One bite too many."	Should have omitted extra helping, or dessert. Feel "heavy" and it's hard to breathe.	Absolutely stuffed; ate and drank enough for two my size; loosen clothing to relieve heavy, tight pressured feeling.	Holidays or celebrations where all-day eating is the occasion. Feel like walking, or sleeping until the heavy, tight feeling subsides.	Out of control consistently. Body is plagued with chronic health risks from long-term overeating.

Caloric Expenditure

Every moment of every day, no matter what activity you engage in, from sleeping to aerobic exercise, you are using up calories. *Caloric energy expenditure is influenced most by how physically active you are all day.* The body's basic needs are more or less fixed, but the amount of physical exertion is a personal decision.

How physically active your life is depends on your choices of profession and recreational activities. It depends upon a multitude of day-to-day choices: whether to walk to the local store or drive the car; use the stairs or elevator; rake the leaves or hire it done; go out for a bicycle ride after supper or watch a TV show. How physically active your life is depends as much on attitude as it does on opportunity.[6]

Figuring Weight Maintenance[7]

1. Record your present weight, in pounds.
2. Record your type of lifestyle. Number values are:
   12 = sedentary
   15 = active physically
   18 = pregnant/nursing
   20 = varsity athlete or physical laborer
3. Multiply (1) × (2).

This is your weight maintenance number, or the number of calories per day you need to eat to *stay* at your current weight.

Caloric Expenditures for Various Activities

How many calories you burn per minute during any activity depends upon two criteria:

1. *Intensity* (high-, medium-, or low-level work or exercise).
2. *Body weight.*

The higher the intensity, the more calories you burn per minute. For example, you expend more energy and calories running a mile than you do walking that mile. The heavier you are, the more calories per minute you will burn (just as full-size cars burn more fuel per mile than small, compact models).

Caloric Intake Needed to Gain Lean Weight

To add one pound of body muscle requires 2,500 calories. (This includes about 600 calories for the muscle and the extra energy needed for exercise to develop the muscle.) Thus, the daily caloric excess, over your maintenance number just figured, is 360.[8] You must be at or below your ideal weight to go on an excess calorie-eating program to gain muscle. You want to use your excess body fat first for your energy requirements.

> *To gain 1 pound of muscle:*
> 2,500 calories equivalent to 1 pound of muscle
> ÷ 7 days in a week
> = 360 daily excess calories to eat over your maintenance intake number

Taking in more than 1,000 calories per day over the number needed to maintain weight, however, is likely to result in weight gain as body fat even if you are exercising strenuously on a regular basis.[9]

Caloric Intake Needed to Lose Body Fat

To lose more than 2 to 3 pounds of body fat per week is physiologically impossible.[10] Weight loss greater than this is in the form of water and lean body tissue. To drop unwanted extra body fat systematically, you need to drop 3,500 calories a week, or 500 per day, to lose one pound of body fat per week.

> *To lose 1 pound fat:*
> 3,500 calories
> ÷ 7 days per week
> = 500 calories a day fewer than your maintenance number

If you desire to drop more pounds per week but the total caloric intake would be less than 1,200, you need to reestablish your goal to lose only 1 pound per week. You never want to eat fewer than 1,200 calories per day. A daily diet of fewer than 1,200 calories is likely to be deficient in needed nutrients for you to grow, repair, stay well, and have energy to perform daily tasks and leisure. Sometimes, on a one-to-one basis, a doctor will have a patient eat fewer than 1,200 calories per day, but will provide extensive guidelines and supplementation. This is *only* under the strict supervision of a doctor.

ESTABLISHING A WEIGHT-WELLNESS MINDSET[11]

Change can be exciting. If you are ready to improve your body composition (lean weight to fat weight ratio) and establish a healthy slimness, change must *begin* at the internal motivational sensory level (see Chapter 2). Assess how you have thought about weight management, eating, and exercising in the past. Is it the "diet-thinking" mentality that is basically *pain*-motivated? Or is it the weight-wellness mindset (Table 14.5), in which pleasures, positives, and possibilities prevail?

Reflect over the following challenges and check where your mindset is now. Goal-set to reframe your thinking and actions to a more positive mindset. These wellness, pleasure-based, motivational pictures, self-talk, and feelings will help you to maintain your lifetime weight management goals.

TABLE 14.5 "Diet" Thinking Versus Weight-Wellness Mindset

"Diet" Thinking	Challenge	Weight-Wellness Mindset
● Any weight loss as measured on scales that society/others think I should lose ● Achieve body image determined by society	GOAL	● Personal self-confidence in my ability to continually make the best choices from available food options ● Wellness/balance is my choice of lifestyle
● Any *rapid* weight loss is acceptable — fat weight OR lean weight	PROGRESS/ PROCESS	● *Gradual* lifestyle changes for the better; conscious awareness of all choices and options
● Overall: negative ● Perfectionistic ● Many limitations and restrictions	ATTITUDE	● Overall: positive ● Flexible; can flow with available options ● Many possibilities/choices available
● Only after achieving weight loss	SELF ACCEPTANCE/ WORTH	● Beginning now, and increasing with each moment of awareness as more distinctions are made
● It's "work" and an unwanted painful necessity ● Confusion: some say I should, some say I shouldn't	EXERCISE	● I enjoy moving as a pleasureable necessity ● It's energizing, fun, and a positive outlet for stress ● Understand it's a required part of the energy formula for proper weight loss/gain
● Slow-moving	SPEED OF MOVEMENT	● Fast-moving
● Negative: food is the enemy; I must deprive myself and use my willpower against desires ● Select only "diet" labels	FOOD	● Food is the friend ● Celebrate! Enjoy, taste, savor each bite ● Creativity of choices and color variety
● Fast (as if this were "the last supper"!) ● Very slow (methodical; avoidance; deceptive)	SPEED OF EATING	● Savoring-paced.
● All-or-nothing approach: "I can eat it all"/ "I can't have any of *that*!"	SELF-TALK	● "I enjoy having it if and when I really choose it. Moderation is my guideline"
● Limited "diet" dictates ● No choices	CHOICE	● I am in charge and I decide what and when to eat. Freedom.
● External ● Blame others/environment frequently/"victim"	CONTROL	● Internal ● Take ownership/"victor"

(continued)

TABLE 14.5 Continued.

"Diet" Thinking	Challenge	Weight-Wellness Mindset
• Don't wait for, or experience, internal cues • Use "appetite" or *mental* cues like the external sensory cues of sight/sound/smell/taste/touch to eat. • May also use distress to trigger eating response like boredom, anxiety, social acceptance, etc.	CUES TO EAT	• *Physical* cues • I am in tune to listen to my body's internal cues for physical hunger like: empty tank; headachy; shakey; "too light;" ready for fuel! • Consider nonfood response to stress like walking, writing, sports, friends.
• Reactionary; • Satisfy now	WILLPOWER	• Proactive: *plan for* various results I choose • Patience, can wait
• *Comfort*, for now • Feel better immediately • Enjoy the "full & heavy" feeling before they stop eating ('6-plus'). Or, "very empty and very light" ("0-2" on dial).	FEELING SENSE	• *Nurturing* for growth and the future. • Know what "satisfied, comfortable, full, yet light" feels like ("5" on dial). Know how much to select, and when to stop eating.
• Needed protection from: neglect; physical or sexual abuse; a low self-image; poor social or coping skills.	BODY FAT VIEWED AS	• Stored energy • Necessary protection of my vital organs.
• Have a *self-prescribed* best way(s) to achieve weight loss • Follow the movie stars' diets	WEIGHT-LOSS PRESCRIPTION	• Follow guidelines and programs from *certified fitness professionals*.
• Avoid pain: Moving-away-from reasons. • *Present* tense in terms of picturing/self-talking/feeling. • "See food" diet: see food and am hungry.	MOTIVATION	• Gain pleasure: moving-toward reasons. • *Future pictures, talk, and feelings.* • "That'll: sit well; give me gas; make me feel just right and satisfied; too full."
• Focused on "diet" they're following; label claims, amount, and caloric value of food before, during, and after eating.	CONVERSATION	• New people, surroundings, and ideas going on.
• Only when goal weight is achieved	SUCCESS DEFINED	• Ideal lean-to-fat ratio for cardiovascular best health — assessed, understood, and worked on through daily living choices in *all* dimensions of life: emotional/social/intellectual/spiritual/talent expression/physical.

"Diet" Thinking	OTHER CHALLENGE	Weight-Wellness Mindset
•	_____	•
•	_____	•
•	_____	•
•	_____	•

Goal Setting Challenge

Set a goal to become more aware of your thinking and actions regarding your body composition or self-image. Set a goal to *achieve* what may be taking up a lot of your mental energy at present. Convert your wishes into small, continual, conscious choices.

Developing Goal Scripts for Chapter 14

DIRECTIONS: Write complete sentences for each segment below. Combine your responses to all four segments. This goal script is designed around your needs and choices. Read it (or make an audiotape and play it) twice daily, morning and evening, until you master it.

1 State one goal in positive, *present-tense* language. Ask yourself, "What will I experience — see, hear, taste, smell, feel — in regard to the results? Keep in mind that all powerful goals use the SMART formula: specific, measurable, achievable, realistic, timely.

_____

_____

2 State your *pleasure-value reasons.* Ask yourself, "Why am I totally committed to achieving this goal? What am I choosing to feel?"

_____

_____

3 State your *pain-avoidance value reasons.* Ask yourself, "What painful values do I choose to avoid feeling?"

_____

_____

4 State *immediate action(s)* you can take in the next 24 hours. Use positive, present-tense verbs such as *choose* and verbs ending with "ing."

_____

_____

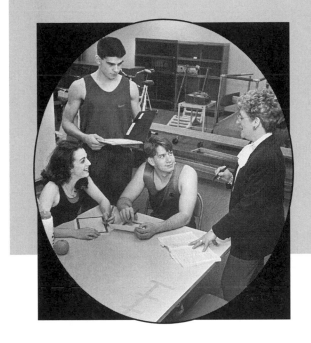

Evaluating Your Fitness Program

As mentioned in the opening chapter of *Fitness Through Aerobics and Step Training*, your total physical fitness program requires:

- making a *commitment* to fitness
- seeking valid *information*
- establishing your *starting points*
- setting reasonable and challenging *goals*

- *monitoring* your daily progress
- making self-disciplined *choices* continually.

This final chapter provides further support for each of these six landmarks in the journeying process. The forms that follow in this chapter are in addition to those presented in each chapter.

CONTENTS

A Commitment To Fitness

I (name) _____ ,

am determined that today (date) _____ ,

am committed to becoming fit!

> I acknowledge that I am in need of improvement in various facets of my well-being (physical, social, emotional, spiritual, intellectual, talent expression) and commit to devote _____ minutes **EVERY** day toward making positive change in my fitness habits. This is in addition to the time spent in class.

> The best time of day for me to work on this change is _____ AM/PM. At this very moment, I am scheduling that daily timeframe on my date book, just for me.

> Absolutely **NOTHING** will take presidence over this block of time that I have set aside to experience personal fitness gains.

Signed _____

Dates: _____
                        (from)   (to)

This commitment
was witnessed by _____ (date) _____

By witnessing this commitment, I am agreeing to be continually supportive and encouraging to this special friend.

*GOALS I'D LIKE TO ACHIEVE DURING THIS COURSE:

1. _____

2. _____

3. _____

4. _____

5. _____

6. _____

7. _____

8. _____

9. _____

10. _____

*As you goal-set the challenges in each chapter, list each one here. This will provide you with a quick reference to the goals you set. Possibly record these on an audiotape, and play it twice daily (morning and night) until these goals are achieved.

GOALS I'D LIKE TO ACHIEVE DURING THIS COURSE:

11. _____

12. _____

13. _____

14. _____

15. _____

16. _____

17. _____

18. _____

19. _____

20. _____

Fitness Journal

DATE	EXERCISE MODE	TIME DURATION	SHORT-TERM GOAL	TODAY'S ACHIEVEMENT	THOUGHTS AND FEELINGS

Fitness Journal

DATE	EXERCISE MODE	TIME DURATION	SHORT-TERM GOAL	TODAY'S ACHIEVEMENT	THOUGHTS AND FEELINGS

Review your fitness journal, detailing your exercise program and the data you kept. Will regular exercise be a lifetime choice?

Target Heart Rates

Record 6-second or 10-second heart rate counts, for the two aerobic intervals that you monitor in class. Were you over or under your target heart rate training zone?

Week	I		II		III		IV		V		VI		VII		VIII		IX		X	
Class	1	2	1	2	1	2	1	2	1	2	1	2	1	2	1	2	1	2	1	2
Aerobic Intervals -1-																				
-2-																				

& Ratings of Perceived Exertion

What did you 'feel' during the various segments of your workout hour?

0.5	very very very light
1	very light
2	light (weak)
3	moderate
4	some-what hard
5	heavy/ strong
6	
7	very hard
8	
9	very very heavy
10	almost maximum

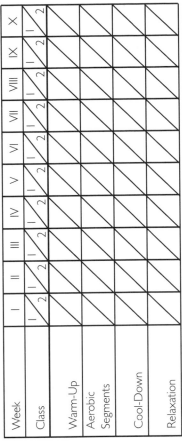

Week	I		II		III		IV		V		VI		VII		VIII		IX		X	
Class	1	2	1	2	1	2	1	2	1	2	1	2	1	2	1	2	1	2	1	2
Warm-Up																				
Aerobic Segments																				
Cool-Down																				
Relaxation																				

Monitoring Your Resting Heart Rate

NOTE: Take your resting heart rate at the first possibility in the A.M., before arising. Use first two fingers at thumb side of wrist, carotid artery in neck, temple area, or other pulse point.

Week	II		III		IV		V		VI		VII		VIII		IX		X	
Class	1	2	1	2	1	2	1	2	1	2	1	2	1	2	1	2	1	2
90 and above																		
85																		
80																		
75																		
70																		
65																		
60																		
55																		
50																		
45																		
40																		
35 and below																		

Bi-Weekly Resting Heart Rate

Resting H.R.—Week 1: _____   At Finish: _____   (—)Loss/(+)Gain: _____

MOTIVATION: "WHAT DO YOU SAY, WHEN YOU TALK TO YOUR SELF?"

STEP I. ASSESSMENT

Have you ever listened to your "intra-personal" communication? We talk to ourselves 100% of our waking hours and our internal dialogue is either positive and enabling, or negative and disabling to us.

What do YOU say when you talk to yourself? Become aware and listen to yourself for an hour, a day, two days, or a week, and write your internal dialogue statements (both positive and negative) as shown in the examples.

Our self-talk usually takes the form of "I" statements followed by: "am / enjoy / hate / fear / think / feel / want / need / worry about /" etc.

Examples:

● "I enjoy Peter and his attention to details."

◉ "I have been such a klutz! I've dropped everything today."

● ●

STEP II. EVALUATION

After you've recorded your Self-Talk for up to one week, go back and evaluate each comment as positive or negative. Circle the ● preceding the comment, if it was *negative* Self-Talk.

Total up those evaluated as positive and negative below.

Totals: + = _____ ; – = _____

STEP III. RE-PROGRAMMING

After awareness, the next step in re-programming a negative disabling attitude expressed through your self-talk is accomplished by updating and actually *re-wording each negative statement* you wrote down so that each reads as positive and enabling to you. This opens a main channel for you to begin to achieve your goal of attitude improvement.

1. A listing of negative language you are replacing includes all of the following *past or future tense verbs and adverbs* (i.e., in regards to personal attitude and fitness mindset improvement): need to, want to, ought to, should, could, wish, used to be, and was.

2. Re-write each of the predicate phrases, using positive, *present-tense* language (I am; I enjoy; I can; and use verbs with "ing" on them as much as possible) and state them *as if you have already achieved the outcome of the new script you're choosing to program.*

Example: **Old:** I need to quit smoking. **New:** "I *enjoy being* a non-smoker."

3. You can *add another* helpful line or two, to each new script, if you wish.

Example: **Old:** I need to cut out eating high fat, high salt, and highly sugared foods like cookies for snacks when I get hungry mid-morning at work. **New:** I enjoy selecting a highly nutritional, low-calorie snack like fruit or juice when I get hungry mid-morning. *I feel better about myself every time I make this better choice.*

4. It is best to state positives of positives. However, if you choose to add the negative because you think it will help, place it as the second or *last sentence* of your new script.

Example: **Old:** I need to exercise more than once a week, and eat less junk food like doughnuts. **New:** I am exercising 3 miles every day and enjoy being a "fat-burner" instead of a "fat-storer." *I never eat FAT PILLS (doughnuts) any more!*

5. Be *specific* as to the outcome of each new scripts' goal. Tell your brain exactly what you want and are now choosing to do.

Example: **Old:** I enjoy exercising to improve my health. **New:** I enjoy exercising for 40 *continuous minutes,* 4 or *more days every week,* to continue achieving my goal of *dropping a pound of body fat a week.*

STEP IV. MAKING YOUR OWN RE-PROGRAMMING-FOR-IMPROVEMENT TAPE

The development of your very own "Tape Talk" tool can prove to be one of the most influential and quickest ways for you to achieve changes you're choosing to make. Here are the details.

1. Purchase a good, blank audiotape cassette that is at least 30 minutes in length on a side. Give it an interesting title!

2. Review your self-management self-talk assessment (Step I) and take note of some of the most used negative self-talk ideas or phrases you use (Steps II). Select 15-18 re-programmed scripts (Step III) to tape.

3. The new programmed scripts you tape can also be re-worded beliefs/ philosophies that you now choose to adopt, that haven't "stuck" yet. Remember to use positive, present tense language throughout.

4. Take your written-out, prepared new scripts, and on the tape, repeat each of the suggestions 3 times, with a short pause in between each suggestion.

5. Repeat this procedure for each new script. (If you have 15 new scripts, there will be a total of 45 suggestions; if you use 18 new suggestions, there will be 54 new suggestions.)

6. End the tape session by recording *each of the phrases/scripts one more additional time each, but this time change "I" to "You."* This provides for the external validation that we all need to have. The total number of scripts on your entire tape will now be the total of 60/72.

Example: "I am a good listener and enjoy hearing what others have to say" becomes... "*You* are a good listener and enjoy hearing what others have to say."

7. If at all possible, add appropriate instrumental music while you tape. Soft, pulsating music seems to affect the way the brain receives and permanently stores information. In order to do this, you'll need an additional tape player, playing the music on it separate from your taping instrument.

8. Talk your scripts onto your tape with emotion! Any programming you currently have in your head is and has been more permanently etched if you experienced it in a highly emotional state.

9. Remember to enjoy reworking your thoughts in language you will enjoy hearing! This is a lot of fun, and just wait until you begin experiencing the results! It is exciting how quickly it can all happen if you are faithful in playing your tape with regularity.

10. Play your tape while you are doing something else — getting ready each morning, during a break while you are relaxing, during a drive in the car to or from class or work, or as you are getting ready for bed. *Play it once or twice a day the first 3 weeks;* then once a day until you realize ... I've mastered these! It's time to make a *new* tape on other new challenges!

MONITORING FOOD AND BEVERAGE INTAKE FOR ONE WEEK

DIRECTIONS: Enjoy recording your food and beverage intake, one day at a time, for one week. It will require just a moment's reflection as you identify the points listed. After one week, ask yourself: "How do my choices measure up to the standards established for a balanced diet, with special attention to selecting nutrient-dense foods?"

● Place a checkmark next to each nutrient-dense food choice you made, on the left, before each food/ beverage entry.

● If you're *really* into qualifying the ratings, identify the rating for each food (4-star/3-star, etc.).

● Comment regarding the social and emotional aspects of your eating patterns.

● Practice the feeling sense and rate 0-10 how "empty"/"full" you feel before, during, and after your meals or snacks.

● Set a goal to improve one aspect of your diet or eating actions that need the most attention.

Food Intake Diary — For One Day

Date:	*Nutrient Density	Name of Food	Food Groups: Ml/Me/V/F/B/SF	How Much	Alone	Family	Friends	Where	Before	During	After	Worried	Bored	Depressed	Tired	Social	Hungry	Other:	How Long (Number of Minutes)	Other Activity While Eating
BREAKFAST																				
SNACK																				
LUNCH																				
SNACK																				
DINNER																				
SNACK																				

Food Intake Diary — For One Day

Date:	*Nutrient Density	Name of Food	Food Groups: Mi/Me/V/F/B/SF	How Much	With Whom			Where	Eating Dial			Why							How Long (Number of Minutes)	Other Activity While Eating
					Alone	Family	Friends		Before	During	After	Worried	Bored	Depressed	Tired	Social	Hungry	Other:		
BREAKFAST																				
SNACK																				
LUNCH																				
SNACK																				
DINNER																				
SNACK																				

Food Intake Diary — For One Day

Date:	*Nutrient Density	Name of Food	Food Groups: Mi/Me/V/F/B/SF	How Much	With Whom			Where	Eating Dial			Why							How Long (Number of Minutes)	Other Activity While Eating
					Alone	Family	Friends		Before	During	After	Worried	Bored	Depressed	Tired	Social	Hungry	Other:		
BREAKFAST																				
SNACK																				
LUNCH																				
SNACK																				
DINNER																				
SNACK																				

Food Intake Diary — For One Day

Date:	*Nutrient Density	Name of Food	Food Groups: Ml/Me/V/F/B/SF	How Much	With Whom			Where	Eating Dial			Why							How Long (Number of Minutes)	Other Activity While Eating
					Alone	Family	Friends		Before	During	After	Worried	Bored	Depressed	Tired	Social	Hungry	Other:		
BREAKFAST																				
SNACK																				
LUNCH																				
SNACK																				
DINNER																				
SNACK																				

Food Intake Diary — For One Day

Date:	*Nutrient Density	Name of Food	Food Groups: Ml/Me/V/F/B/SF	How Much	With Whom			Where	Eating Dial			Why							How Long (Number of Minutes)	Other Activity While Eating
					Alone	Family	Friends		Before	During	After	Worried	Bored	Depressed	Tired	Social	Hungry	Other:		
BREAKFAST																				
SNACK																				
LUNCH																				
SNACK																				
DINNER																				
SNACK																				

Food Intake Diary — For One Day

Date:	*Nutrient Density	Name of Food	Food Groups: Mi/Me/V/F/B/SF	How Much	With Whom			Where	Eating Dial			Why							How Long (Number of Minutes)	Other Activity While Eating
					Alone	Family	Friends		Before	During	After	Worried	Bored	Depressed	Tired	Social	Hungry	Other:		
BREAKFAST																				
SNACK																				
LUNCH																				
SNACK																				
DINNER																				
SNACK																				

Food Intake Diary — For One Day

Date:	*Nutrient Density	Name of Food	Food Groups: Mi/Me/V/F/B/SF	How Much	With Whom			Where	Eating Dial			Why							How Long (Number of Minutes)	Other Activity While Eating
					Alone	Family	Friends		Before	During	After	Worried	Bored	Depressed	Tired	Social	Hungry	Other:		
BREAKFAST																				
SNACK																				
LUNCH																				
SNACK																				
DINNER																				
SNACK																				

FITNESS COURSE SELF-ASSESSMENT CHECK SHEET

Techniques / Skills / Knowledge

DIRECTIONS: In preparation for your practical and written final examination, go over each key point listed, and practice each technique and skill given. This self-evaluation instrument can be a valuable tool for future use.

KEY:

- 4 / A = always
- 3 / U = usually
- 2 / O = occasionally
- 1 / S = seldom
- 0 / N = never

Aerobics

- Know how to determine resting heart rate.
- Know how to determine target heart rate.
- Warm-up exercises are active, medium to low level, rhythmic, limbering, standing, full range of motion.
- Perform slow, sustained static stretching (no bounce).
- Engage in continuous breathing.
- Exhale during stretch: inhale as release from stretch.
- During low-impact: legs kept low, arms below heart.
- During power low-impact: hip, knee, ankle extending moves are followed by a knee flexion, ankle-springing action; one foot always in contact with the floor; space is well used.
- During high/low-impact: higher knees performed and arms overhead more frequently; both airborne and grounded moves are used.
- During low-impact cool-down: active, rhythmic, full range of motion, but low-level, slower, half-tempo moves are performed.
- Post-aerobic stretching includes: standing stretches for hamstrings, quadriceps, and calves.
- Know how to vary intensity and impacts.

Step Training

- Know how to select proper bench height.
- Use proper posture: keep back straight, head and chest up, shoulders back, abdomen tight and buttocks tucked under hips.
- Lean forward slightly with the whole body. Don't bend at hips.
- Step up lightly, making sure whole foot lands on platform.
- Do not lock knees when stepping up.
- Step down close to platform, not back.
- Bring heel down to floor before taking next step.
- Avoid excess arm movements over head.
- Maintain appropriate speed for safe movement.
- Do not pivot or twist on weight-bearing leg.
- Maintain muscular balance by working opposing muscle groups.
- Know bench/step directional approaches / orientations.
- Can perform single lead base step.
- Can perform alternating lead base step.
- Can perform step touch (w/bench tap, floor tap lunge).
- Can perform v-step.
- Can perform straddle down.

Techniques / Skills / Knowledge

KEY:

- 4 / A = always
- 3 / U = usually
- 2 / O = occasionally
- 1 / S = seldom
- 0 / N = never

Step Training (cont.)

- Can perform straddle up.
- Can perform single and alternating bypass moves (knee, kick back, side leg lift).
- Can perform lunge (from side and end).
- Can perform turn step.
- Can perform over the top.
- Can perform repeaters.
- Can perform propulsion steps.
- Limit propulsions and power moves.
- Can perform single skill sequence (change one element at a time).
- Can perform double skill sequence.
- Can perform multiple skill sequence.

Strength

- Precede strength training with static stretching.
- Joints and spine are stabilized before each exercise.
- Smooth, continuous, full range of motion movements performed.
- Maintain slow timing and are not jerky.
- Take 2 seconds to overcome resistance.
- Take 2 to 4 seconds during release/lowering resistance.
- Exhale during lifting phase; inhale during lowering phase.
- Visualization and self-talk are engaged.
- 1-3 sets, 8-12 reps format.
- Can add 1-4 lbs. resistance.
- Brief rest period is taken between bouts.
- Can lift and lower whole body against gravity.
- Can properly add weight resistance to body part used.
- Can control use of hand-held weights.
- Can use rubber resistance bands efficiently and effectively.
- Can use rubber resistance tubing efficiently and effectively.
- Can combine tubing with bench workout.
- Can combine step with strength using tubing and the bench in intervals of 3 min. step, to 1 min. strength-with-tubing.

Flexibility

- Can actively stretch slowly, with position held at joint extreme.
- Can gently press slowly beyond this point without motion.
- Can mentally relax, visualize, self-talk and hold for 15 seconds.
- Can withdraw slowly from stretch.
- Perform to opposite side of body for each stretch.
- Can perform at least one PNF stretch.

Relaxation

- Can construct powerful images to relax.
- Can construct positive self-talk affirmations.
- Can deep-breathe and effectively lower after-workout heart rate.

Total Fitness Course Post-Assessment

Take a moment and reflect upon what you've learned and the personal progress you've made. Review all of the fitness assessments you completed during the course. From which assessment did you gain the most insight about yourself and your ability to make choices?

Review these Post-Assessment questions to identify and quantify any change that has occurred.

1 Did you keep a regular time commitment (dates with yourself) to work on your program outside of class?

2 Regarding your motivation:

Are you usually motivated *toward pleasure* or to *avoid pain*?

Which sense is most vital to *your* learning — visual/auditory/kinesthetic?

3 Retake a laboratory physical fitness test ("stress test"): Cooper's 12-Minute or 1.5-Mile Run/ Walk Test, or Cooper's 3-Mile Walking Test.

What is your present fitness level (category/ quantified times and distances)?

What change have you experienced over the past 10 (or so) weeks?

4 What was your initial resting heart rate?

What is it now?

What key occurrences this term have resulted in *significant* raising/lowering of your resting heart rate?

5 How many days per week did you do:

Stretching exercises?	Duration?
Aerobics?	Duration?
Step training?	Duration?
Fitness walking?	Duration?
Alternative aerobic exercises?	Duration?
Strength training?	Duration?
Relaxation techniques?	Duration?

6 What exercise prescription do you plan to continue weekly?

7 What are your favorite forms of stress release?

8 What positive changes have you made in your quest for managing your total well-being (besides Physical):

Emotionally?

Socially?

Spiritually?

Intellectually?

Expressing your talents?

9 What is your heart rate after 3 minutes of relaxation?
How does this compare to your current resting heart rate?

10 Have a post-assessment body composition evaluation performed (another 3-site skinfold measurement).

Has your lean weight increased or decreased?

Has your fat weight increased or decreased?

Your present weight "category" is:

11 Take a look at your daily and weekly consumption of food and beverage. Have you improved your food and beverage intake?

Is it now more nutritionally balanced since the assessment was first made?

12 What do you need to ensure a lifetime fitness commitment?

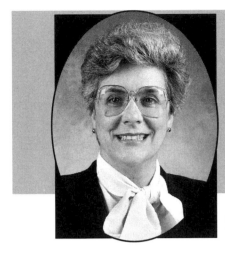

Notes

Karen S. Mazzeo, M.Ed.
Educator • Author • Consultant

CHAPTER 1

1. Terry W. Parsons, "Positive Lifestyle Strategies," lecture quoting Kenneth Cooper's research in Anchor Fitness Course, September 18, 1990.
2. Kenneth H. Cooper, "Run Dick, Run Jane," (Provo, UT: Brigham Young University, 1971) (Film).
3. Kenneth H. Cooper, *The Aerobics Way* (New York: M. Evans and Company, 1977), p. 10.
4. National Vital Statistics Division, National Center for Health Statistics, Rockville, MD, 1994.
5. American College of Sports Medicine 1990: Position Stand, "The Recommended Quality and Quantity of Exercise for Developing and Maintaining Cardiorespiratory and Muscular Fitness in Healthy Adults," *Medical Science Sports Exercise,* 22(2), (1990), pp. 265– 274.
6. Lenore R. Zohman et al., *The Cardiologists' Guide to Fitness and Health Through Exercise* (New York: Simon and Schuster, 1979), p. 72.
7. *Harvard Medical School Health Letter,* 10(6) (April 1985), p. 3.
8. Harvard.
9. Harvard.
10. ACSM Position Stand, 1990.
11. ACSM.
12. ACSM.
13. ACSM.
14. ACSM.
15. Unpublished research data by Karen S. Mazzeo collected on students enrolled in aerobic dance courses, 1984–1986.
16. G. A. V. Borg, "Psychophysical Bases of Perceived Exertion," *Medicine and Science in Sport and Exercise* 14 (1982).
17. Charlotte A. Williams, "THR Versus RPE: The Debate Over Monitoring Exercise Intensity," *IDEA Today,* April 1991, p. 42.
18. Williams, p. 42.

CHAPTER 2

1. Bernie Rabin, Ed.D, educational and clinical psychologist, yearly guest speaker to Karen S. Mazzeo's Tension Management and Health Methods courses, Bowling Green State University, 1978–1988.
2. Shad Helmstetter *What To Say When You Talk to Yourself* (New York: Pocket Books/Simon & Schuster, 1986), p. 98.
3. Karen S. Mazzeo, *Stress*Time* Life Management* Principles, Methods, and Assessment Techniques* (Bowling Green, OH: Mazzeo Reprographics, 1995) p. 42.

4. Anthony Robbins, *Unlimited Power* (New York: Fawcett/ Columbine 1986), pp. 125–148.
5. Connirae Andreas et al., *Heart of the Mind* (Moab, UT: Real People Press, 1989), pp. 254–255.
6. Robert Dilts et al., *Neuro-Linguistic Programming: The Study of the Structure of Subjective Experience* (Cupertino, CA: Meta Publications, 1980).
7. David Gordeon et al., *The Neuro-Linguistic Programming Home Study Guide* (San Rafael, CA: FuturePace).

CHAPTER 3

1. Lenore Zohman et al., *The Cardiologists' Guide to Fitness and Health Through Exercise* (New York: Simon and Schuster, 1979), p. 81.
2. Zohman.
3. American College of Obstetricians and Gynecologists, *Safety Guidelines for Women Who Exercise* (ACOG Home Exercise Programs No. 2). Washington DC: ACOG, 1986), p. 6.
4. Douglas H. Richie, Jr. "How to Choose Shoes," *IDEA Today,* April 1991, p. 67.
5. Richie.
6. ACOG, p. 5.
7. ACOG, pp. 4–5.
8. Orthotic for sports shoe prescribed and dispensed by Dr. Charles Marlowe, podiatrist to Karen S. Mazzeo, summer 1983.
9. ACOG, No. 2, p. 5.
10. Committee on Nutritional Misinformation, Food and Nutrition Board, National Research Council, National Academy of Sciences, "Water Deprivation and Performance of Athletics," distributed by Nutritional Education and Training Program, Bowling Green State University, 1981.
11. American Alliance for Health, Physical Education, and Recreation, *Nutrition for Athletes. A Handbook for Coaches* (Washington, DC: AAHPERD, 1971), p. 42.
12. AAHPERD, *Nutrition for Sport Success* (Reston, VA: AAHPERD), 1984, p. 2.
13. American College of Sports Medicine, *Encyclopedia of Sports Sciences and Medicine* (New York: Macmillan, 1971), p. 215.
14. ACSM, p. 216.
15. ACSM, p. 216.
16. Interview with Jane Steinberg, athletic trainer of intercollegiate sports, Bowling Green State University, Bowling Green, Ohio, spring 1982.
17. ACOG, p. 6.
18. Interview, Steinberg, 1982.

19. Harvard Medical School Health Letter, 11 (5), p. 4.

CHAPTER 5

1. Kenneth H. Cooper, *Running Without Fear* (New York: M. Evans and Company, 1985), p. 128.
2. Cooper, p. 192.
3. Cooper, p. 197.
4. Cooper, *The Aerobics Program for Total Well Being* (New York: M. Evans and Company, 1982), pp. 141–142.
5. Lenore R. Zohman et al., *The Cardiologists' Guide to Fitness and Health Through Exercise* (New York: Simon and Schuster, 1979), p. 87.

CHAPTER 6

1. Candace Copeland-Brooks, *Moves... and More!* (San Diego: IDEA, Inc. 1990). (videotape)
2. Copeland, *The Low-Impact Challenge for the Fitness Professional* (Newark, NJ: PPI Entertainment Group/Parade Video, 1991). (videotape)
3. Julie Moo-Bradley and Jerrie Moo-Thurman, *Aerobics Choreography in Action: The High-Low Impact Advantage.* (San Diego: IDEA, Inc. 1990). (videotape)
4. Lynne Brick, *Total Body Workout* (Philadelphia: Creative Instructors Aerobics, 1991). (videotape)
5. Amy Jones, "Point-Counterpoint: Sequencing a Dance-Exercise Class," *Dance Exercise Today,* May/June 1985.
6. American College of Obstetricians and Gynecologists, *Safety Guidelines for Women Who Exercise* (ACOG Home Exercise Programs) (Washington, DC: ACOG, 1986).
7. James L. Hesson, *Weight Training for Life* (Englewood, CO: Morton Publishing, 1985).
8. SPRI Products, 1554 Barclay Blvd., Buffalo Grove, IL 60089, *Pumping Rubber* (instructions for product use), 1988, 1-800-222-7774).
9. John Patrick O'Shea, *Scientific Principles and Methods of Strength Fitness,* 2d ed. (Reading, MA: Addison-Wesley, 1976).
10. Len Kravitz et al., "Static & PNF Stretches," *IDEA Today,* March 1990.

CHAPTER 7

1. Ken Alan, "A Choreography Primer," *IDEA Today,* January 1989.
2. Lorna Francis et al., "Moderate-Impact Aerobics," *IDEA Today,* September 1989.

3. Lorna Francis et al., "Injury Prevention. Low-Impact Aerobics: 'Do's and Don'ts." *Dance Exercise Today*, Nov./Dec. 1986.
4. Alan.
5. Francis, Lorna et al. "Moderate-Impact Aerobics."
6. Francis, "Injury Prevention."
7. Francis, "Moderate-Impact Aerobics." Also, *Aerobics Choreography* (San Diego: IDEA, Association for Fitness Professionals, 1990).
8. Candace Copeland, *The Low-Impact Challenge for the Fitness Professional* (Newark, NJ: PPI Entertainment Group/Parade Video, 1991). (videotape)
9. Francis, "Moderate-Impact Aerobics."
10. Copeland videotape, 1991.
11. Francis, "Moderate-Impact Aerobics," 1989.
12. Francis.
13. Francis.
14. "Research: Caloric Expenditure in LIA vs HIA" from study, 'The Metabolic Cost of Instructor's Low Impact and High Impact Aerobic Dance Sequences,' *IDEA Today*, January 1991, p. 8.
15. "Tempo and Ground Reaction Forces for LIA and HIA," from study 'Comparison of Forces in High and Low Impact Aerobic Dance at Various Tempos,' *IDEA Today*, May 1991, p. 9.
16. IDEA, *Aerobics Choreography* (San Diego: IDEA: Association for Fitness Professionals, 1989).
17. Karen S. Mazzeo et al., *Aerobic Dance — A Way to Fitness*, 2d ed. (Englewood, CO: Morton Publishing, 1987), p. 112.
18. Mazzeo, 113.

CHAPTER 8

1. Joan Price, "Stepping Basics," *IDEA Today*, November/December 1990, p. 57.
2. Len Kravitz and Rich Deivert, "The Safe Way To Step," *IDEA Today*, April 1991.
3. Sports Step, Inc. *Introduction to Step Training*, (Atlanta: 1989). (videotape)
4. Lynne Brick and David Essel, *Pump n' Step* (1991). (videotape)
5. Lorna Francis, Peter Francis, and Gin Miller, *Step-Reebok. The First Aerobic Training Workout with Muscle. Instructor Training Manual* (Reebok International, 1990).
6. Francis.
7. Len Kravitz, "The Safe Way To Step." *IDEA Today*, April 1991, pp. 47–50.
8. D. Stanforth et al., "The Effect of Bench Height and Rate of Stepping on the Metabolic Cost of Bench Stepping," *Medicine and Science in Sport and Exercise* (abstract), 23(4) (April 1991), S143.
9. Francis, p. 17.
10. Francis, p. 23.
11. Francis, pp. 23–25.
12. Francis.
13. Francis.
14. Francis.
15. Francis.
16. Sports Step, Inc., videotape accompanying *The Step: Introduction to Step Training* (Atlanta, Sports Step, 1989).
17. Karen S. Mazzeo and Lauren M. Mangili, *Instructor's Manual for Step Training Plus* (Englewood, CO: Morton Publishing, 1993) p. 33. (Adapted for this textbook)

CHAPTER 9

1. Kenneth H. Cooper, *The Aerobics Program for Total Well-Being* (New York: M. Evans and Company, 1982), p. 129.
2. Cooper, p. 144.

3. Level I Walking Only Program was written by Dr. Richard W. Bowers, ACSM-certified program director, Fitwell Program, Student Recreation Center, Bowling Green State University, Bowling Green, Ohio, 1990.
4. Steven N. Blair, *Exercise and Health: Sports Science Exchange,* (Gatorade Sports Science Institute, November 1990) (Vol. 3, #29).
5. Kathleen Hargarten, "A Rope-Jumping Class," *IDEA Today*, March 1989.

CHAPTER 10

1. American College of Obstetricians and Gynecologists, *Safety Guidelines for Women Who Exercise* (ACOG Home Exercise Programs) (Washington, DC: ACOG, 1986), p. 6.
2. James L. Hesson, *Weight Training for Life* (Englewood, CO: Morton Publishing, 1985), p. 33.
3. Hesson.
4. Sports Step, Inc. Videotape accompanying *The Step, Introduction to Step Training* (Atlanta: Sports Step, 1989).
5. SPRI Products, Inc., *Pumping Rubber* (instructions for product use) (Buffalo Grove, IL, 1988).
6. SPRI.
7. SPRI.
8. SPRI.
9. American College of Sports Medicine: Position Stand, "The Recommended Quality and Quantity of Exercise for Developing and Maintaining Cardiorespiratory and Muscular Fitness in Healthy Adults," *Medical Science Sports Exercise* 22:2 (1990), pp. 265–274.
10. Hesson, pp. 164–165.
11. SPRI.
12. Lynn Brick and David Eassel, Pump n' Step (1991). (videotape)
13. SPRI Products, Inc. and Brick Bodies, *Step Strength* (Buffalo Grove, IL: SPRI Products).
14. John Patrick O'Shea, *Scientific Principles and Methods of Strength Fitness*, 2nd ed (Reading, MA: Addison-Wesley, 1976), p. 89.

CHAPTER 11

1. Len Kravitz et al., "Static & PNF Stretches," *IDEA Today*, March 1990.
2. Kravitz et al.
3. Kravitz et al.
4. Kravitz et al.

CHAPTER 12

1. John S. J. Power, *Why Am I Afraid to Tell You Who I Am?* (Allen, TX: Tabor Publishing, 1969), p. 56.
2. Hans Selye, *Stress Without Distress* (Toronto: McClelland and Stewart Limited, 1974), p. 141.
3. Roman Carek, Director of the Counseling and Career Development Center, Bowling Green State University, Bowling Green, Ohio, from his stress management presentation in the LIFE Seminar Workshop Series, 1982, held at the Student Recreation Center of BGSU.
4. Taken in part from technique developed by Dr. Bernie Rabin, psychologist and lecturer to Karen Mazzeo's Personal Wellness, Health Methods, and Stress Management classes 1980–1988, Bowling Green State University, Bowling Green, Ohio.
5. Adapted from an original "Natural Highs" model, given to Karen Mazzeo's Personal Wellness class, Bowling Green State University, Bowling Green, Ohio, 1988, by an anonymous student.
6. Rabin, 1988.

CHAPTER 13

1. Nutrition Education Services. *"Pyramid Plus, A Star-Studded Guide to Food Choices for Better Health"*, (Portland, Oregon Dairy Council, 1994).
2. Judy Tillapaugh, "Cross-Training in the Kitchen," *IDEA Today*, October, 1991, p. 21.
3. U. S. Department of Agriculture, *Food Guide Pyramid, A Guide to Daily Food Choices* (Washington, DC: U.S. Government Printing Office 1992).
4. Nutrition Education Services/ Oregon Dairy Council, "Pyramid Plus" pamphlet.
5. Nutrition Education Services.
6. Nutrition Education Services.
7. National Dairy Council, "Guide to Wise Food Choices" B 170-1 (Rosemont, IL: National Dairy Council, 1978), p. 1.
8. Nutrition Education Services.
9. Nutrition Education Services.
10. U. S. Department of Agriculture, Human Nutrition Information Service, Home & Garden Bulletin No. 253-2, p. 5, July 1993 (Washington, DC: Government Printing Office).
11. USDA, Home & Garden Bulletin Numbers 253-1 through 253-8.
12. Jan Lewis, "Nutrition Notes: Nutrition and the Athlete" Workshop Series, Nutrition Education and Training Program, Bowling Green State University, Bowling Green, OH, 1981.
13. USDA, Home & Garden Bulletin Numbers 253–1 through 253–8.
14. Lucy M. Williams, lecture and literature, "Shopping Tips for Low Fat, Low Salt, Low Cholesterol Diets," delivered to Karen S. Mazzeo's Anchor Fitness-Personal Excellence class, February, 1991.
15. Williams.
16. USDA, Home & Garden Bulletin Number 253–8, p. 2.
17. U. S. Department of Agriculture, Food Safety and Inspection Service, "An Introduction to the New Food Label," DHHS Publication NO (FDA) 94–2271, USDA FSIS–41, October 1993.

CHAPTER 14

1. Werner W. K. Hoeger, *Principles & Labs for Physical Fitness & Wellness* (Englewood, CO Morton Publishing, 1994), pp. 49–64.
2. Jan Lewis, "Nutrition Notes. Dietary Guidelines 2," Bowling Green State University, Bowling Green, OH, 1981.
3. Dr. Steven Blair, keynote speaker at 1992 American Alliance for Health, Physical Education, Recreation, & Dance National Convention, Indianapolis, IN.
4. Connirae Andreas and Steven A. Andreas, *Heart of the Mind* (Moab, UT: Real People Press, 1989), p. 251.
5. Andreas, p. 125.
6. Lewis, p. 6.
7. Kenneth H. Cooper, *The Aerobics Way* (New York: M. Evans and Company, 1977), p. 142.
8. Lewis, p. 4.
9. Lewis.
10. Lewis.
11. Tammy Kime-Sheets and Karen S. Mazzeo, "Establishing A Weight-Wellness Mindset," methods pamphlet and instructional tool given during presentations to Bowling Green State University, Ohio students in Tension Management Classes, and professional seminars for clients, Spring, 1995.

Index

Note: Boldfaced entries refer to actual exercises or illustrations.